Klavdija Čuček Trifkovič, Mateja Lorber, Nataša Mlinar Reljić, Gregor Štiglic (Eds.)
Innovative Nursing Care

Innovative Nursing Care

Education and Research

Edited by
Klavdija Čuček Trifkovič, Mateja Lorber,
Nataša Mlinar Reljić, Gregor Štiglic

DE GRUYTER

Editors

Klavdija Čuček Trifkovič, PhD, RN
Žitna ulica 15
SI-2000 Maribor
Slovenia
klavdija.cucek@um.si

Mateja Lorber, PhD, RN
Žitna ulica 15
SI-2000 Maribor
Slovenia
mateja.lorber@um.si

Nataša Mlinar Reljić, PhD, RN
Žitna ulica 15
SI-2000 Maribor
Slovenia
natasa.mlinar@um.si

Gregor Štiglic, PhD, RN
Žitna ulica 15
SI-2000 Maribor
Slovenia
gregor.stiglic@um.si

ISBN 978-3-11-078592-0
e-ISBN (PDF) 978-3-11-078608-8
e-ISBN (EPUB) 978-3-11-078617-0
DOI https://doi.org/10.1515/9783110786088

Library of Congress Control Number: 2022947490

Bibliographic information published by the Deutsche Nationalbibliothek
The Deutsche Nationalbibliothek lists this publication in the Deutsche Nationalbibliografie;
detailed bibliographic data are available on the internet at http://dnb.dnb.de.

Cover image: gpointstudio/iStock/Getty Images Plus
Typesetting: Integra Software Services Pvt. Ltd.
Printing and binding: CPI books GmbH, Leck

www.degruyter.com

Preface

People are living longer than ever before which may be partly ascribed to improved healthcare literacy. However, increasing lifespan also increases the complexity of nursing and general health care problems. This makes providing optimal nursing care even more challenging and increases the significance of nurses' education.

Insufficient education and knowledge can lead to errors in nursing care; therefore, improving knowledge is vital for delivering quality nursing care. Education and awareness of best nursing practice care delivery include devotion to being a professional, being up to date, striving to improve, and ultimately providing the finest nursing care to people, families, and communities.

Research assists nurses in determining best practice and enhancing nursing care. Additionally, nursing research assists in adapting to changes in the present healthcare environment, patient demographics, and legal requirements. As researchers uncover new findings, the nursing practice continues to evolve.

This book aims to contribute to creative nursing care in the larger field of nursing and will thus be valuable to nurses and nursing students in a variety of nursing specialties. It is structured into the following three sections: Clinical nursing; Holistic nursing care; and Education in nursing. The first section consists of six chapters demonstrating different methodological approaches used on examples ranging from capturing the experiences of parents in during the pandemic using a cross-sectional approach to a review of mobile applications. In the second section on holistic nursing, again under six chapters, a wide range of methodological approaches is presented and demonstrated in different fields of nursing, from capturing ethical issues in palliative care to measuring the caring processes. The final section consists of three chapters focusing on nursing students and the educational process.

We would like to express our gratitude to all the reviewers who contributed to multiple improvements in the final versions of the chapters. Additionally, we would like to thank Professor Roger Watson for language editing as well as Gregor Romih and Zvonka Fekonja, who were overseeing the review process. It is also difficult to imagine preparing this book without Jessika Kischke from deGruyter, who kindly guided us through the editorial process.

Klavdija Čuček Trifkovič, Mateja Lorber, Nataša Mlinar Reljić and Gregor Štiglic

Contents

List of Contributors

Assistant Professor Amanda Briggs, RN, MSc
School of Nursing and Healthcare Leadership
University of Bradford
Bradford, UK
a.briggs4@bradford.ac.uk
Chapter 6

Teaching Assistant Leona Cilar Budler,
PhD, RN
Faculty of Health Sciences
University of Maribor
Žitna ulica 15
2000 Maribor, Slovenia
leona.cilar1@um.si
Chapters 1, 3, 6, 14, 15

Senior Lecturer Klavdija Čuček Trifkovič,
PhD, RN
Faculty of Health Sciences
University of Maribor
Žitna ulica 15
2000 Maribor, Slovenia
klavdija.cucek@um.si
Chapters 3, 6, 14

Suzanne Denieffe, PhD
School of Humanities
Waterford Institute of Technology
Waterford, Ireland
sdenieffe@wit.ie
Chapter 14

Assistant Professor Margaret Denny, PhD
Faculty of Health Sciences
University of Maribor
Žitna ulica 15
2000 Maribor, Slovenia
denny.margaret@gmail.com
Chapter 14

Assistant Professor Mojca Dobnik, PhD, RN
Ministry of Health
Štefanova ulica 5
1000 Ljubljana, Slovenia
mojcadobnik@hotmail.com
Chapter 5

Senior Lecturer Barbara Donik, RN, BSc, MSc
Faculty of Health Sciences
University of Maribor
Žitna ulica 15
2000 Maribor, Slovenia
barbara.donik@um.si
Chapter 7

Urška Fekonja, RN
University Medical Centre Maribor
Ljubljanska ulica 5
2000 Maribor, Slovenia
urska.fekonja1@student.um.si
Chapters 7, 9

Teaching Assistant Zvonka Fekonja, RN, BSc
Faculty of Health Sciences
University of Maribor
Žitna ulica 15
2000 Maribor, Slovenia
zvonka.fekonja@um.si
Chapters 2, 7, 8, 9, 10, 11

Teaching Assistant Nino Fijačko, RN
Faculty of Health Sciences
University of Maribor
Žitna ulica 15
2000 Maribor, Slovenia
nino.fijacko@um.si
Chapter 6

Senior Lecturer Vida Gönc, RN, BSc, MSc
Faculty of Health Sciences
University of Maribor
Žitna ulica 15
2000 Maribor, Slovenia
vida.goenc@um.si
Chapter 10

Teaching Assistant Lucija Gosak, RN
Faculty of Health Sciences
University of Maribor
Žitna ulica 15
2000 Maribor, Slovenia
lucija.gosak2@um.si
Chapter 6

Principal Lecturer Irma Mikkonen, PhD, MNSc
Savonia University of Applied Sciences
Finland
Chapter 7

Sabina Herle
Društvo za avtizem DAN
Finžgarjeva 21
2000 Maribor, Slovenia
sabina.herle@siol.net
Chapter 3

Senior Lecturer Barbara Kegl, RN, BSc, MSc
Faculty of Health Sciences,
University of Maribor
Žitna ulica 15
2000 Maribor, Slovenia
barbara.kegl@um.si
Chapters 1, 8

Teaching Assistant Petra Klanjšek, RN
Faculty of Health Sciences
University of Maribor
Žitna ulica 15
2000 Maribor, Slovenia
petra.klanjsek@um.si
Chapter 1

Teaching Assistant Sergej Kmetec, RN
Faculty of Health Sciences
University of Maribor
Žitna ulica 15
2000 Maribor, Slovenia
sergej.kmetec1@um.si
Chapters 2, 3, 7, 8, 9, 10, 11

Primož Kocbek, BSc
Faculty of Health Sciences
University of Maribor
Žitna ulica 15
2000 Maribor, Slovenia
primoz.kocbek@um.si
Chapter 13

Professor Blanka Kores Plesničar, PhD, MD
University Psychiatric Clinic Ljubljana
Chengdujska 45
1260 Ljubljana, Slovenia
blanka.kores@psih-klinika.si
Chapter 11

Kathy Leadbitter, PhD
Division of Neuroscience and Experimental
Psychology
University of Manchester
Manchester
UK
Kathy.Leadbitter@manchester.ac.uk
Chapter 3

Associate Professor Mateja Lorber, PhD, RN
Faculty of Health Sciences
University of Maribor
Žitna ulica 15
2000 Maribor, Slovenia
mateja.lorber@um.si
Chapters 5, 9

Urša Markež, RN
University Medical Centre Maribor
Ljubljanska ulica 5
2000 Maribor, Slovenia
ursa.markez@student.um.si
Chapter 9

Professor Tracy McClelland, PhD, RN
School of Nursing and Healthcare Leadership
University of Bradford
Bradford, UK
g.t.mcclelland@bradford.ac.uk
Chapter 6

Professor Brendan McCormack, DPhil
(Oxon.), BSc (Hons.), PGCEA, RGN, RMN,
FRCN, FEANS
School of Health Sciences
Queen Margaret University Edinburgh
Musselburgh, UK
bmccormack@qmu.ac.uk
Chapters 2, 8, 9, 10

Assistant Professor Nataša Mlinar Reljić,
PhD, RN
Faculty of Health Sciences
University of Maribor
Žitna ulica 15
2000 Maribor, Slovenia
natasa.mlinar@um.si
Chapters 7, 8, 11

Teaching Assistant Kasandra Musović, RN
Faculty of Health Sciences
University of Maribor
Žitna ulica 15
2000 Maribor, Slovenia
kasandra.musovic1@um.si
Chapters 13, 14

John Nelson, PhD, MS, RN
Healthcare Environment
St Paul
MN, USA
john@healthcareenvironment.com
Chapter 12

Lecturer Jasmina Nerat, RN, BSc
Faculty of Health Sciences
University of Maribor
Žitna ulica 15
2000 Maribor, Slovenia
jasmina.nerat@um.si
Chapter 2

Professor Dušica Pahor, PhD, MD
Faculty of Medicine
University of Maribor
Taborska ulica 8
2000 Maribor, Slovenia
dusica.pahor@um.si
Chapter 4

Professor Majda Pajnkihar, PhD, RN, FAAN,
FEANS
Faculty of Health Sciences
University of Maribor
Žitna ulica 15
2000 Maribor, Slovenia
majda.pajnkihar@um.si
Chapters 4, 11, 12, 13

Rok Perkič, RN
University Medical Centre Maribor
Ljubljanska ulica 5
2000 Maribor, Slovenia
Chapter 2

Lecturer Tatjana Ribič, RN, BSc, MSc
SeneCura Nursing Home Maribor
Cesta Osvobodilne fronte 43
2000 Maribor, Slovenia
tatjana.ribic@soncnidom.si
Chapter 11

Professor Jackie Rowles, DNP, MBA, MA,
CRNA, ANP-BC, FNAP, FAAP
Texas Christian University School of Nurse
Anesthesia
Fort Worth, TX, USA
j.rowles@tcu.edu
Chapter 5

Assistant Professor Tara L. Sacco, PhD, RN
Wegmans School of Nursing
St. John Fisher College
3690 East ave
Rochester, NY 14618, USA
tsacco@sjfc.edu
Chapter 1

Professor Marlaine Smith, PhD, RN, AHN-BC,
HWNC-BC, FAAN
Christine E. Lynn College of Nursing
Florida Atlantic University
Boca Raton, FL, USA
msmit230@health.fau.edu
Chapter 13

Lecturer Marija Spevan, RN, MSc
Faculty of Health Studies
University of Rijeka
Viktora Cara Emina 5
51000 Rijeka, Croatia
mspevan@fzsri.uniri.hr
Chapter 14

Associate Professor Gregor Štiglic, PhD
Faculty of Health Sciences
University of Maribor
Žitna ulica 15
2000 Maribor, Slovenia
and
Faculty of Electrical Engineering and
Computer Science
University of Maribor
Koroška cesta 46
2000 Maribor, Slovenia
and
Usher Institute
University of Edinburgh
Edinburgh, UK
gregor.stiglic@um.si
Chapters 3, 6, 13, 14, 15

Associate Professor Jadranka Stričević,
PhD, RN
Faculty of Health Sciences
University of Maribor
Žitna ulica 15
2000 Maribor, Slovenia
jadranka.stricevic@um.si
Chapter 1

Associate Professor Matej Strnad, PhD, MD
University Medical Centre Maribor
Ljubljanska ulica 5
2000 Maribor, Slovenia
matej.strnad@um.si
Chapters 2, 9

Professor Fiona Timmins, PhD
School of Nursing, Midwifery and Health
Systems
University College Dublin
Dublin, Ireland
fiona.timmins@ucd.ie
Chapter 11

Assistant Professor Dominika Vrbnjak,
PhD, RN
Faculty of Health Sciences
University of Maribor
Žitna ulica 15
2000 Maribor, Slovenia
dominika.vrbnjak@um.si
Chapters 4, 12, 13

Professor Roger Watson, PhD, RN, FAAN
Usher Institute
University of Edinburgh
Edinburgh, UK
and
Faculty of Health Sciences
School of Health and Social Work
University of Hull
Hull, UK
rwatson1955@gmail.com
Chapter 15

Petra Klanjšek, Leona Cilar Budler, Jadranka Stričević,
Tara L. Sacco, Barbara Kegl

1 Parents experiences in Slovenia during the COVID-19 pandemic

Abstract

Introduction: The COVID-19 pandemic emerged here in March 2020. The pandemic and lockdowns have been the cause of many parents doing both paid and unpaid work at home. Everyday life was a great challenge. Challenges, insecurities, and changes have caused people anxiety and fear, which has been and will only be reflected in the mental well-being of individuals. We wanted to find out how parents faced their fears, worries, and daily lives during the epidemic.

Methods: A cross-sectional study was conducted to gain insight into parents' experiences during the COVID-19 pandemic in Slovenia. Casual parental sampling was used and a total of 135 parents participated. To collect data, we developed a questionnaire based on a literature review. In addition, mental well-being was measured using the Warwick-Edinburgh Mental Well-being scale. Finally, the results were analysed in the SPSS and R programs with the help of descriptive and inferential statistics.

Results: We found that 26.0% of children had SARS-CoV-2 and that few parents worked from home; 85.0% had the opportunity to provide protective equipment to all family members. Parents and children were dissatisfied with the change of life during the epidemic; children mainly due to the lack of social contacts. Of parents 74.0% spent more time with their children due to the lockdown and 56.0% had to be substitute teachers for their children using distance learning. The most common fear was that the adults would bring the infection home and get sick, the child would get hurt, or the parent would get sick. Parental mental well-being was average ($M = 53.20$; $SD = 9.61$) and did not differ between the sexes ($p > 0.05$).

Discussion: We found that parents were most afraid of bringing the infection into the home environment. Parents had to provide care and assistance to their children while working at home or at work. They had to do more unpaid work in the family and were more mentally burdened. Parents were more burdened and dissatisfied with the change of life, but they quickly adapted to these circumstances, so their mental well-being remained unchanged. The children were disappointed with the ban on socializing with their peers and distance learning.

Conclusion: With the duration of the pandemic, people were more afraid of changed life circumstances and worries about work, care, and schooling of children than they were of the infection. Despite the gradual release of measures to limit the spread of COVID-19, people still followed self-protection measures. Now, however, due to unclear information, people are confused when and where it is necessary to take protective measures. A pandemic is a process that takes a long time, so real consequences will be shown with delay. We believe that, given the rapid spread of various viruses around the world, we will have to adapt to this different life and face the challenges posed by pandemics in the future.

Keywords: coronavirus, impact, mental well-being, children

1.1 Introduction

The COVID-19 pandemic has affected people across the globe [1]. In Slovenia, the first infection with the new coronavirus was confirmed on 4 March 2020 [2]. On 11 March 2020, the World Health Organization (WHO) classified COVID-19 as a global pandemic as the virus spreads across more than 100 countries [3]. As a result, schools and some employers transitioned to virtual settings [4]. Nearly 90.0% of adults ($n = 11,537$) reported that their lives had changed since the COVID-19 epidemic, with 44.0% indicating a significant change [4]. Also, in Slovenia, children and students were educated at home from 16 March 2020 until June 2020 [5] and then also from 15 October 2020 to 1 February 2021 [6] when the youngest children (6–8 years old) first returned to school. During this time, kindergartens were also closed [5]. At the same time, sports activities were banned; these regulations began to relax on 12 April 2021 [7].

During the COVID-19 pandemic, the parents coordinated their work, family, and school responsibilities. Because of this, parents introduced new rules and faced different challenges in the dynamics of the family, such as teaching children, school assignments, and social distancing [8]. In addition, there were differences between families in dealing with problems and challenges according to the age of the children, the workload of the parents, and the lower paid work [1, 9].

A stable and secure environment is essential for optimal child development. The children need routine because that way, they know what to expect. Breaking the routine and changes are significant stressors that negatively affect a child's sense of security [10, 11] and the whole family's safety [12]. Parental tasks increased significantly during the COVID-19 pandemic: stay at home, taking care of the children 24 h a day, taking care of the education of their children, started working from home, working outside the regular schedule, and some parents also lost their jobs during that time [1, 13]. The stress that parents experienced during the pandemic is associated with psychological, behavioural, and emotional problems in children and adolescents [14–16].

Despite the difficulties and challenges, some parents also reported the positive side of the COVID-19 pandemic, as, during this period, the families spent more time together [17]. On the other hand, the COVID-19 pandemic brings a variety of fears and concerns to people worldwide. Moreover, additional challenges were posed by measures to limit the spread of coronavirus [18, 19], reflecting a decline in human well-being [18] and increase in mental health problems [20], manifested in stress, depression, and anxiety [21–23]. Therefore, we wanted to examine how COVID-19 pandemic and lockdown impacted parents' and children's well-being.

1.2 Methods

1.2.1 Study design

A cross-sectional study was conducted between 1 April 2021 and 1 June 2021.

1.2.2 Participants

The survey was conducted among the adult population of parents in Slovenia. We used a convenience sample that we accessed via the web and social media (e.g., Facebook, LinkedIn, Instagram, and e-mail). We anticipated that the sample would include over 100 individuals. The sample included individuals who voluntarily consented to participate and submitted their answers in an online survey. Before conducting the survey, participants were informed about the purpose of the survey, rights, anonymity, volunteering, and the possibility of withdrawal at any stage of completing the questionnaire. The decision to participate in the study was left entirely to the participants.

1.2.3 Measures

We developed a questionnaire consisted of five parts: (1) demographic questions (who is fulfilling the questionnaire – mother or father; age; education level; study; the number of children; the number of school-aged children; the age of the youngest child; employment status; etc.); (2) questions related to COVID-19 (e.g., if they, their family members, or essential others got the coronavirus; measures taken to prevent COVID-19 infection; child's feeling during COVID-19 pandemic); (3) measures during COVID-19 (e.g., measures to contain the virus and parents fears); (4) immunization and testing (e.g., parents opinion on mandatory children immunization and children testing); and (5) parents mental well-being. The first four parts were developed based on the extensive literature search, analysis, and synthesis. The fifth part consisted of questions in the Warwick-Edinburg Mental Well-being Scale (WEMWBS) [24]. The WEMWBS was developed in Scotland in 2006 and translated in 2017 for use among Slovenian and Northern Ireland nursing students [25, 26].

1.2.4 Data analyses

Using descriptive statistics, we described the sample's demographic characteristics by means of averages, frequencies, and percentages. Then, correlations between variables were tested using inferential statistics. Finally, data were analysed using the statistical programs SPSS and R. The results are presented with the help of tables, graphs, and figures.

1.3 Results

In our study, a total of 111 (79.9%) mothers and 24 (17.3%) fathers fulfilled the questionnaire ($n = 135$). All participants did not answer all questions; thus, the number of participants in individual answers may differ. On average, participants were 40.64 years old (SD = 6.81). A minority ($n = 16$, 11.5%) of participants stated that they are still involved in formal education. The education level of the involved participants is presented in Tab. 1.1.

Tab. 1.1: Education level of involved parents.

Education level	n	%
PhD	8	5.8
Master	17	12.2
University	36	25.9
Higher school	10	7.2
Higher professional school	29	20.9
Secondary school	34	24.5

n, number; %, per cent.

Parents were asked about their salary during the COVID-19 pandemic. About 74.8% ($n = 95$) claimed that they received 100.0% of their salary, 7.9% ($n = 10$) got 80.0% of their salary, and a minority claimed other (e.g., sick leave, pension, and unemployed). We also asked them if they could afford all family members' protections (e.g., masks and gloves). About 95.3% ($n = 121$) answered positively. Other questions and parent's answers are presented in Tab. 1.2.

Also, parents were asked if their children were disappointed with the changed life due to the COVID-19 pandemic. Parents reported that their children were disappointed during the COVID-19 pandemic due to lack of socializing ($n = 25$, 19.7%) and un-attending kindergarten or school ($n = 18$, 14.2%).

Tab. 1.2: COVID-19 related questions.

Questions	Answers	
	Yes n (%)	No n (%)
Did you have COVID-19?	28 (22.0)	96 (75.6)
Did any of your family members had COVID-19?	41 (32.3)	83 (65.4)
Did any of your children had COVID-19?	33 (26.0)	91 (71.7)

n, number; %, per cent.

Of parents 74.0% (n = 94) stated that they spent more time with their children during the COVID-19 pandemic than usual, and 56.7% (n = 72) said that their school-age children needed help from them in gaining new knowledge and homework during the COVID-19 pandemic. Parents also had fears due to COVID-19. The most common parents' answers are presented in Tab. 1.3.

Tab. 1.3: Parents' fears related to COVID-19.

	n	%
That I will lose my job.	1	0.8
That they will take away too many rights that we will never get back.	1	0.8
That we will have no more income.	8	6.3
To infect the elderly.	1	0.8
To infect someone close (grandmother, grandfather).	1	0.8
To infect the older members of family.	1	0.8
To carry the infection home.	52	40.9
That I get hurt.	1	0.8
That the children are getting hurt.	8	6.3
That a child who already has known previous health problems gets worse.	5	3.9
That this madness will never end, but that the world and Slovenian economies will collapse, and we will feel the consequences.	1	0.8
To make a child sick.	23	18.1
To make parents sick.	1	0.8
To make me sick.	8	6.3

n, number; %, per cent.

Parents mainly were afraid that they would bring COVID-19 to their homes, would make their children sick, that their children would get hurt, that they would get sick, and that they would have no income.

At the end of the questionnaire, parents were asked to evaluate all claims related to their mental well-being in the past two weeks. Mental well-being was measured using the WEMWBS scale consisted of 14 items (marked as W1–W14). Parents evaluated claims from 1, meaning never, to 5, meaning always. The minimum score of mental well-being was 29, and the maximum was 70. The higher WEMWBS score the higher the ones' mental well-being. The mean value was 53.20 (SD = 9.61). Mean values for all items and differences between mother and father are shown in Tab. 1.4.

Tab. 1.4: Item and scale scores by mother and father.

Scale item	Mother M (SD)	Father M (SD)
W1	3.78 (0.99)	3.57 (1.03)
W2	3.96 (0.91)	4.00 (0.89)
W3	3.47 (0.90)	3.57 (1.12)
W4	3.74 (0.98)	3.38 (1.16)
W5	3.68 (1.07)	3.38 (1.20)
W6	3.71 (0.89)	3.90 (0.89)
W7	3.90 (0.89)	3.90 (0.89)
W8	3.73 (0.87)	3.95 (1.02)
W9	3.45 (1.03)	3.29 (1.31)
W10	3.89 (0.92)	4.05 (0.81)
W11	4.15 (0.85)	4.14 (0.79)
W12	4.01 (1.03)	4.19 (1.03)
W13	4.03 (0.99)	4.10 (0.89)
W14	3.79 (0.88)	3.95 (1.02)
WEMWBS score	53.27 (9.64)	53.38 (10.27)

M, mean value; SD, standard deviation; WEMWBS, The Warwick-Edinburgh Mental Well-being Scale.

The difference in parental mental well-being is minimum. That is also evident from the box plot (Fig. 1.1).

Data distribution by gender of parents was not normal; thus, non-parametric tests were used when comparing results by gender of parents. Finally, we checked any correlation between parents' mental well-being and their age and refuted this hypothesis ($r(127) = -0.067$, $p = 0.471$).

There was also no correlation between parent mental well-being and number of children ($r(127) = 0.150$, $p = 0.098$) or number of school aged children ($r(127) = 0.085$, $p = 0.369$).

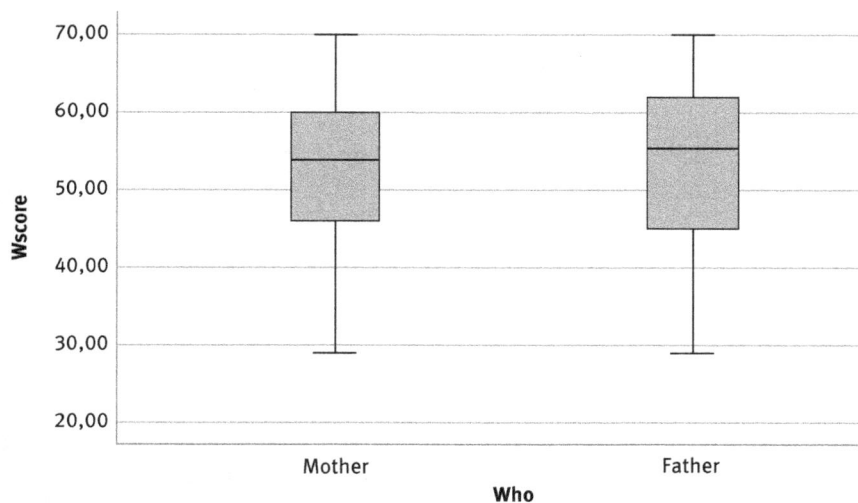

Fig. 1.1: Parental mental well-being.

Parents were asked to evaluate their children's feelings during the COVID-19 pandemic. Their answers are presented in Tab. 1.5. A total of 17.91% of children were in good mood. On the contrary, 44.03% of children were bored. Followed by good mood (38.06%), no will (13.44%), and stubborn (11.94%). Rarely, however, parents reported cheerful (8.21%), verbally rude (8.21%), aggressive (3.73%), and bad will (1.50%). In addition to the above, parents also stated bad mood (11.19%), fun (5.22%), unchanged (3.73%), reluctant (1.50%), and one case for each: good mood, boring at times, but we devoted more time to each other, depending on the day, mood swings, he was not feeling the same the whole time of the pandemic, good-natured, bad-tempered, adolescent (Tab. 1.5).

Also, parents were asked to evaluate their feelings during COVID-19; 25.39% of parents stated that they were in goodwill, 16.42% were in a bad mood, 16.42% were bored, 21.65% of parents indicated that they felt unchanged, and 23.13% had no enthusiasm. Other answers are presented in Tab. 1.5.

Tab. 1.5: Child's and parent's feelings during COVID-19 pandemic.

	Child		Parent	
	n	%	n	%
Bored	59	44.03	22	16.42
Good mood	51	38.06	34	25.39

Tab. 1.5 (continued)

	Child		Parent	
	n	%	n	%
No will	18	13.44	31	23.13
Cheerful	11	8.21	8	6.02
Bad will	2	1.50	7	5.22
Aggressive	5	3.73	4	3.01
Verbally rude	11	8.21	2	1.50
Stubborn	16	11.94	4	3.01
Other answers				
Bad mood	15	11.19	22	16.42
Fun	7	5.22	1	0.75
Unchanged	5	3.73	29	21.65
Reluctant	2	1.50	1	0.75
Good mood	1	0.75	–	–
Boring at times, but we devoted more time to each other	1	0.75	–	–
Depending on the day	1	0.75	–	–
Mood swings	1	0.75	–	–
He wasn't feeling the same the whole time of the epidemic	1	0.75	–	–
Good-natured	1	0.75	–	–
Bad-tempered	1	0.75	–	–
Adolescent	1	0.75	–	–
Overworked	–	–	1	0.75
Overloaded	–	–	2	1.50
Tired	–	–	6	7.46
Weak will	–	–	5	3.73
Nervous	–	–	1	0.75
No matter the situation okay	–	–	1	0.75
See above			1	0.75
Adapted to the situation we accepted	–	–	1	0.75

Tab. 1.5 (continued)

	Child		Parent	
	n	%	n	%
Very good at the beginning, but after a couple of months of combining work and school, the nervousness grew. That is when I decided to wait for childcare.	–	–	1	0.75
The epidemic continues	–	–	1	0.75
It was exhausting	–	–	1	0.75
Stressed and numb	–	–	1	0.75
Every day is different	–	–	1	0.75
All little by little	–	–	1	0.75

n, number; %, per cent.

1.4 Discussion

The outbreak of the COVID-19 pandemic severely affected families with children in Slovenia. We found out that 22.0% of parents, 41.0% of family members, and 26.0% of children got COVID-19. Gassman-Pines et al. [27] reported that in the United States of America, only 12.0% got of families COVID-19. The spread of the infection with SARS-CoV-2 and the adoption of protective measures has changed society and made it difficult to accept the health and economic consequences of the closure of the country. Our results clearly show that the crisis has influenced the psychological well-being of adults and children. The changes happened in a matter of weeks and lasted for more than a year. Parents have reported a deterioration and their children's psychological well-being since the start of the COVID-19 pandemic. This finding is like findings from previous economic crisis studies, which reveal that mental health deteriorates as the country's economic situation deteriorates [28, 29].

A low level of infection with SARS-CoV-2 was detected; consequently, there was no concern among people in the first week of the COVID-19 pandemic in Slovenia. Emotional responses changed just a few days after the first official confirmed case of infection with SARS-CoV-2, which were reflected in concerns about the virus, infection, and thinking about the disease [9]. Negative emotions increased extremely quickly after the onset of the epidemic, and the escalation of events continues to affect the emotional experience [30]. The COVID-19 pandemic has caused people psychological distress (fear, anxiety), in addition to social and economic stress [31]. Also, in our study, we found that parents were mostly afraid to bring the infection home to make a child sick/injured or to get sick themselves. Similar feeling was found by authors in their studies [27, 31]. Parents and children live in stress, fear, and media hype [32] and become insecure and impatient, which represents a challenge for long-term planning [32, 33]. As a result of the state of emergency during the closure of schools, violence against children has increased, and as a result, there have been more reports of child abuse [32].

Due to the closure of Slovenia, childcare, schooling, and in some industries, work has been transferred to the home environment [9, 34]. In our study parents reported that their children were disappointed during the COVID-19 pandemic due to lack of socializing and un-attending kindergarten or school. Parents should help children overcome emotional problems caused by the inability to meet friends [34]. School closures cause problems for students, parents, and teachers [35]. Parents in our study reported about their children's feelings during COVID-19. Only 38.06% of the children and 25.39% parents were in good mood and cheerful. The other children felt bored, no enthusiasm, stubborn, verbally rude, and in a bad mood, according to the parents.

We also found fear of lower monthly incomes, even though in our survey, as many as three-quarters of parents received a 100.0% salary. Also [8] stated that 92.0% of parents maintained employment during the COVID-19 pandemic. We found out that 7.9% of parents stayed at home because schools or kindergarten closed, and they have only 80.0% of salary.

Some parents had to navigate between different roles at home (educator, teacher, etc.). Others went to work daily (shopkeepers, health workers, cleaners, postmen, etc.) with changed and extended working hours, or as usual, exposing themselves to infection risk and at the same time providing care for children at home [1, 34]. During this time, more mothers than fathers worked from home. Mothers also took care of their children at home while working remotely, while fathers usually worked in the office and spent less time with childcare at home. COVID-19 has inevitably increased the inequality of the childcare burden [36, 37]. The parents felt socially isolated, helpless, and insecure due to the lockdown, which poses risks to their well-being [38]. The children of the parents who were at home with their families were more satisfied than the children of the parents who went to work every day [39]. We found that those parents who navigated well between different roles at home were more satisfied, and consequently, the children were also more satisfied.

In our survey, respondents stated that their mental well-being was average. The mean score of parent's mental well-being was 53.20 (SD = 9.61). There were no significant differences in mental well-being by gender, and scores were not correlated to parents' age ($p > 0.05$). Although there are no deviations in parents' mental well-being, attention needs to be paid to the mental well-being of children and parents to reduce the consequences of the COVID-19 pandemic [17, 38], as the daily negative mood of parents affects the mental health of all family members [16, 27, 40]. Children and adolescents need to have access to multidisciplinary professionals in support centres that care for good mental health [40]. In national survey conducted in the USA, 27.0% of parents reported worsening mental health for themselves and 14.0%

reported worsening mental health of children. This is a consequence of loss of regular childcare, change in insurance status, and worsening food security [41]. Also, Gassman-Pines et al. [27] reported that the COVID-19 pandemic significantly worsened parents' and children's psychological well-being. Similar results, indicating worsening parental mental well-being, have been reported by Huebener et al. [42].

1.4.1 Limitations

This study presents parents' opinions on the COVID-19 pandemic in Slovenia and its impact on themselves and their children. Although there is not enough study performed in Slovenia during COVID-19 and its impact on parents and children, this study has some limitations. First, a cross-sectional study was conducted to get insight into parents' opinions on COVID-19 and its impact on child's and parent's mental well-being. To obtain more reliable results, mental well-being should be measured over several time periods. Also, we cannot claim if parent's mental well-being changed during the COVID-19 pandemic. Data were collected using a questionnaire developed by the authors based on current knowledge and literature review. The WEMWBS scale is a self-reporting scale, which means that parents evaluated their mental well-being subjectively. There is a possibility that they gave socially desirable answers. Also, a relatively small sample was included in this study. Due to non-normally distributed data, non-parametric statistical tests were used. Data were collected online using social networks; thus, people who are not using social networks did not have an opportunity to participate in this study. All limitations need to be considered when interpreting the results.

1.5 Conclusion

COVID-19 has dynamically altered several families. Infectious diseases, such as the virus SARS-CoV-2, can disturb the environment in which children grow and develop. Troubled relations inside the family, as well with friends, have negative effects on the entire society as well as on the well-being, development, and protection of the children. Quarantine and isolation rules have a negative effect on the children as well as on their families.

Families in the entire world adapted to the changes and challenges that happened because of the COVID-19 pandemic. For many parents, as well as entire families, it is important to combine work activities with the children's needs. Even though the isolation can be a once in a lifetime opportunity for spending time together and developing relations with our children, many parents and caretakers have different opinions, and problems while adapting, making decisions, and setting-up priorities while battling the pandemic, in addition to finding different ways to form their every-day lives and making them as normal as possible.

References

[1]   Weaver JL, Swank JM. Parents' lived experiences with the COVID-19 pandemic. Family J, 2021, 29(2), 136–142.
[2]   Koronavirus (SARS-CoV-2). Ljubljana: Urad Vlade Republike Slovenije za komuniciranje, (2022. Accessed March 7, 2022, at https://www.gov.si/teme/koronavirus-sars-cov-2/.)
[3]   WHO Director-General's opening remarks at the media briefing on COVID-19-1 February 2022, (2022. Accessed March 7, 2022, at https://www.who.int/director-general/speeches/detail/who-director-general-s-opening-remarks-at-the-media-briefing-on-covid-19—1-february-2022.)
[4]   Most Americans Say Coronavirus Outbreak Has Impacted Their Lives 2020. Washington, DC.: Pew Research Center, (2022. Accessed March 7, 2022, at https://www.pewresearch.org/so cial-trends/2020/03/30/most-americans-say-coronavirus-outbreak-has-impacted-their-lives/)
[5]   Posebno obvestilo ministrice dr. Simone Kustec o varstvu otrok 2020. Ljubljana: Ministrstvo za izobraževanje, znanost in šport, 2020. (Accessed March 6, 2022, at https://www.gov.si/novice/2020-03-15-posebno-obvestilo-ministrice-dr-simone-kustec-o-varstvu-otrok/)
[6]   Križaj M, Pristavec Đogić M, Eror A. Šolanje v času COVID-19: Primerjalni pregled (PP). Ljubljana, Republika Slovenija Državni Zbor, 2021. Accessed March 6, 2022, at https://fotogalerija.dz-rs.si/datoteke/Publikacije/Zborniki_RN/2021/Solanje_v_casu_COVID-19.pdf).
[7]   Nujno obvestilo – Vrtci 2020. Ljubljana: Republika Slovenija GOV.SI, 2020 (Accessed March 6, 2022, at https://www.gov.si/novice/2020-10-23-nujno-obvestilo-vrtci/)
[8]   Craig L, Churchill B. Dual-earner parent couples' work and care during COVID-19. Gend Work Organ, 2020, 28, 66–79.
[9]   Lep Ž, Hacin Beyazoglu K. Psihologija pandemije: Posamezniki in družba v času koronske krize. Ljubljana, Slovenia, Znanstvena založba Filozofske fakultete, 2020, 53–65.
[10]   Fiese BH, Tomcho TJ, Douglas M, Josephs K, Poltrock S, Baker T. A review of 50 years of research on naturally occurring family routines and rituals: Cause for celebration?. J Fam Psychol, 2002, 16, 381–390.
[11]   Sandstrom H, Huerta S. The negative effects of instability on child development: A research synthesis. 2013. (Accessed March 6, 2022, at https://www.urban.org/research/publication/negative-effects-instability-child-development-research-synthesis)
[12]   Prime H, Wade M, Browne DT. Risk and resilience in family well-being during the COVID-19 pandemic. Am Psychol, 2020, 75(5), 631–643.
[13]   Griffith AK. Parental burnout and child maltreatment during the COVID-19 pandemic. J Fam Violence, 2020, 1–7.
[14]   Jiao WY, Wang LN, Liu J, Fang SF, Jiao FY, Pettoello-Mantovani M, et al. Behavioral and emotional disorders in children during the COVID-19 epidemic. J Pediatr, 2020, 221, 264–266.e1.
[15]   Romero E, López-Romero L, Domínguez-Álvarez B, Villar P, Gómez-Fraguela JA. Testing the effects of COVID-19 confinement in Spanish children: The role of parents' distress, emotional problems and specific parenting. Int J Environ Res Public Health, 2020, 17(19), 6975.
[16]   Spinelli A, Pellino G. COVID-19 pandemic: Perspectives on an unfolding crisis. Br J Surg, 2020, 107(7), 785–787.

[17] Fontanesi L, Marchetti D, Mazza C, Di Giandomenico S, Roma P, Verrocchio MC. The effect of the COVID-19 lockdown on parents: A call to adopt urgent measures. Psychol Trauma, 2020, 12(S1), S79–S81.

[18] Zacher H, Rudolph CW. Individual differences and changes in subjective wellbeing during the early stages of the COVID-19 pandemic. Am Psychol, 2021, 76(1), 50–62.

[19] Bavel JJV, Baicker K, Boggio PS, Capraro V, Cichocka A, Cikara M, et al. Using social and behavioural science to support COVID-19 pandemic response. Nat Hum Behav, 2020, 4(5), 460–471.

[20] Chandola T, Kumari M, Booker CL, Benzeval M. The mental health impact of COVID-19 and lockdown-related stressors among adults in the UK. Psychol Med, 2020, 1–10.

[21] Casagrande M, Favieri F, Tambelli R, Forte G. The enemy who sealed the world: Effects quarantine due to the COVID-19 on sleep quality, anxiety, and psychological distress in the Italian population. Sleep Med, 2020, 75, 12–20.

[22] Odriozola-González P, Planchuelo-Gómez Á, Irurtia MJ, de Luis-garcía R. Psychological effects of the COVID-19 outbreak and lockdown among students and workers of a Spanish university. Psychiatry Res, 2020, 290, 113108.

[23] Petzold MB, Bendau A, Plag J, Pyrkosch L, Mascarell Maricic L, Betzler F, et al. Risk, resilience, psychological distress, and anxiety at the beginning of the COVID-19 pandemic in Germany. Brain Behav, 2020, 10(9), e01745.

[24] Tennant R, Hiller L, Fishwick R, Platt S, Joseph S, Weich S, et al. The Warwick-Edinburgh Mental Well-Being Scale (WEMWBS): Development and UK validation. Health Qual Life Outcomes, 2007, 5, 63.

[25] Cilar L, Štiglic G, Kmetec S, Barr O, Pajnkihar M. Effectiveness of school-based mental well-being interventions among adolescents: A systematic review. J Adv Nurs, 2020, 76(8), 2023–2045.

[26] Cilar L, Barr O, Štiglic G, Pajnkihar M. Mental well-being among nursing students in Slovenia and Northern Ireland: A survey. Nurse Educ Pract, 2019, 39, 130–135.

[27] Gassman-Pines A, Ananat EO, Fitz-Henley J. COVID-19 and parent-child psychological well-being. Pediatrics, 2020, 146(4), e2020007294.

[28] Gassman-Pines A, Ananat EO, Gibson-Davis CM. Effects of statewide job losses on adolescent suicide-related behaviors. Am J Public Health, 2014, 104(10), 1964–1970.

[29] Ananat EO, Gassman-Pines A, Francis DV, Gibson-Davis CM. Linking job loss, inequality, mental health, and education. Science, 2017, 356(6343), 1127–1128.

[30] Wang H, Xia Q, Xiong Z, Li Z, Xiang W, Yuan Y, Liu Y, et al. The psychological distress and coping styles in the early stages of the 2019 coronavirus disease (COVID-19) epidemic in the general mainland Chinese population: A web-based survey. PloS One, 2020, 15(5), e0233410.

[31] Darlington AE, Morgan JE, Wagland R, Sodergren SC, Culliford D, Gamble A, et al. COVID-19 and children with cancer: Parents' experiences, anxieties and support needs. Pediatr Blood Cancer, 2021, 68(2), e28790.

[32] Cluver L, Lachman JM, Sherr L, Wessels I, Krug E, Rakotomalala S, et al. Parenting in a time of COVID-19. Lancet, 2020, 395(10231), e64.

[33] Janssen LHC, Kullberg MJ, Verkuil B, van Zwieten N, Wever MCM, van Houtum L, et al. Does the COVID-19 pandemic impact parents' and adolescents' well-being? An EMA-study on daily affect and parenting. PloS One, 2020, 15(10), e0240962.

[34] Daniela L, Rubene Z, Rūdolfa A. Parents' perspectives on remote learning in the pandemic context. Sustainability, 2021, 13(7), 3640.

[35] Tadesse S, Muluye W. The impact of COVID-19 pandemic on education system in developing countries: A review. Open J Soc Sci, 2020, 8(10), 159–170.

[36] Yamamura E, Tsustsui Y. The impact of closing schools on working from home during the COVID-19 pandemic: Evidence using panel data from Japan. Rev Econ Househ, 2021, 19(1), 41–60.

[37] Dong C, Cao S, Li H. Young children's online learning during COVID-19 pandemic: Chinese parents' beliefs and attitudes. Child Youth Serv Rev, 2020, 118, 105440.

[38] Cusinato M, Iannattone S, Spoto A, Poli M, Moretti C, Gatta M, et al. Stress, resilience, and well-being in Italian children and their parents during the COVID-19 pandemic. Int J Environ Res Public Health, 2020, 17(22), 8297.

[39] Maheshwari S, Mehndiratta S. Parental outlook and problems faced during lockdown in COVID-19 pandemic: Experience from a paediatric haematology-oncology unit in a developing country-A questionnaire-based survey. J Clin Diagn Res, 2021, 15(4), 1–4.

[40] Singh S, Roy D, Sinha K, Parveen S, Sharma G, Joshi G. Impact of COVID-19 and lockdown on mental health of children and adolescents: A narrative review with recommendations. Psychiatry Res, 2020, 293, 113429.

[41] Patrick SW, Henkhaus LE, Zickafoose JS, Lovell K, Halvorson A, Loch S, et al. Well-being of parents and children during the COVID-19 pandemic: A national survey. Pediatrics, 2020, 146(4), e2020016824.

[42] Huebener M, Waights S, Spiess CK, Siegel NA, Wagner GG. Parental well-being in times of Covid-19 in Germany. Rev Econ Househ, 2021, 1–32.

Zvonka Fekonja, Rok Perkič, Matej Strnad, Sergej Kmetec,
Brendan McCormack

2 Symptoms experienced by patients with acute myocardial infarction that the triage nurses should know in the emergency department: a systematic review

Abstract

Background: Vascular and heart disease present a big problem in public health society. Acute myocardial infarction (AMI), which belongs under acute coronary syndromes, is one of the most common diseases and biggest causes of early death in developed countries. Symptoms in patients with myocardial infarction vary between typical and atypical symptoms. This review aims to identify different AMI symptoms of patients who seek medical attention in the emergency department (ED).

Methods: A systematic review of the literature in CINAHL, MEDLINE, ScienceDirect, and SAGE was conducted to identify studies on detected symptoms in patients with myocardial infarction over 18 years in the ED. The search was limited to studies on this topic published up to December 2021. The data analysis was based on thematic analysis.

Results: Out of 2,814 studies retrieved, 11 studies were included. The data analysis identified one main theme: clinical symptoms and three subcategories.

Conclusion: The triage nurses need to pay attention to cardiovascular symptoms, such as chest pain, the most common symptom. Their focus also needs to be redirected to epigastric pain and cold sweating, which are abdominal and systemic symptoms, and anxiety and nausea/vomiting in patients with diabetes.

Impact: AMI is one of the most common diseases and causes of early death in developed countries. The literature lacks knowledge about the different symptoms of AMI, which the triage nurses must be careful about. The knowledge and rapid identification of myocardial infarction helps triage nurses provide the best outcomes.

Keywords: acute coronary syndrome, emergency department, myocardial infarction, review

2.1 Introduction

Cardiovascular conditions are the most frequent cause of death in Europe, representing 45% of all deaths, 49% of female deaths, and 40% of male deaths [1]. Acute myocardial infarction (AMI) is the most common and important form of ischemic cardiac disease and falls under acute coronary syndrome (ACS) [2]. ACS develops because of erosion or rupture of atherosclerosis plaque in the coronary artery by which a blood clot is formed. The blood clot partially or entirely blocks the lumen in coronary arteries, leading to the heart muscle's ischemia. Long-lasting ischemia leads to an AMI; however, blood clots are the leading cause of myocardial infarction [3].

AMI can manifest itself in two ways, namely with ST-segment elevation (STEMI) or without ST-segment elevation (NSTEMI) [4]. The symptoms of myocardial infarction may be hard to distinguish clinically. Therefore, the diagnosis can be verified only by electrocardiography, elevated blood biomarkers, or radiological diagnostics [5]. The most common cardinal symptom when dealing with AMI is chest pain [6].

In addition, it is well known that certain groups of patients (e.g., women, older patients, and individuals with diabetes) [7–10] do not always have chest pain and experience fewer characteristic symptoms [7]. The nonspecific symptoms of AMI could be found by history taking or physical examination and are presented as fatigue, shortness of breath, pain in the back, neck, arm or upper abdomen, oedema, and nausea [11]. Furthermore, Thygesen et al. [12] describes nonspecific symptoms of ischemia of the myocardium as uncomfortable pressure in the chest, upper extremities, and jaw. The diagnosis could incorrectly be identified and often confused with gastrointestinal, neurological, pulmonary, or musculoskeletal diseases because of these symptoms [13].

The emergency department (ED) is the first point of contact for many patients seeking help [14]. Once the patient arrives at the ED, the first step is triage. In triage, a nurse assesses the patient's condition and asks the patient a series of questions about their main complaints, medical history, the clinical presentation of the symptoms, transportation mode, the presence and time-frame of pain in the chest area, and the patient's general appearance [15, 16]. The measurement of vital signs such as body temperature, heart rate, respiratory rate, blood pressure, and pulse oximetry is considered a standard part of the triage examination. All that information determines the patient's appropriate triage category [17]. The accuracy of nurses' triage decisions, based on their experience, knowledge, perceptions, and intuition to achieve the quickest medical evaluation, electrocardiogram (ECG) recording, and interpretation of that record within 10 min of arrival to the ED, are potential interventions that could save the patient's life [18].

However, triage nurses can sometimes overlook the AMI symptoms because of the patient's appearance and clinical signs, especially when presented with AMI's atypical or nonspecific clinical signs [19]. In such cases, the triage nurse could evaluate a patient's symptoms as other diseases, and the patient may not receive timely treatment [20]. Moreover, in one kind of AMI (NSTEMI), there are typically no changes in the ECG, and patients do not present with AMI's typical signs and symptoms [21]. Consequently, triage nurses should rely not only on the empirical data but also on their attitudes, experiences, intuition, and intuition when dealing with AMI and in decision-making for further health care and treatment of those patients [22].

Many studies have been focused either on symptoms of potential ACSs or conducted to measure different demographic factors such as gender, race, and other variables separately [23]. Therefore, the chapter aims to identify what symptoms a triage nurse needs to know in patients with suspected AMI in an ED.

2.2 Methods

A systematic review was conducted following the methodology and recommendations of Preferred Reporting Items for Systematic Reviews (PRISMA) [24]. This methodological approach allows analysis, knowledge synthesis, and applicability of the results to practice. The process of searching and data extraction of the studies was guided by the PRISMA [24] guidelines and is presented in the flow diagram (Fig. 2.1).

2.2.1 Research question

For the systematic review, we developed a PIO question: Among patients with AMI who are seeking help at the ED (P), which signs and symptoms (I) are identified by triage nurses (O)?

2.2.2 Search strategy

We conducted a systematic review in CINAHL, MEDLINE, SAGE, and ScienceDirect databases using the search terms in English: AMI, symptoms, signs, emergency, and triage nurses, including their synonyms and Boolean operators (AND/OR). The posed limitations were research papers in English relating to the research topic without a set timespan.

2.2.3 Review approach and selection criteria

Inclusion criteria for the selection of papers were: (1) adult person with diagnosed AMI; (2) seeking help at the ED; (3) research papers that used quantitative, qualitative, and mixed-methods research approaches; and (4) identifying signs and symptoms of AMI. Exclusion criteria were: (1) adult person without diagnosed AMI, (2) not seeking help at the ED; (3) papers that used systematic review as a research methodology or other types of reviews of the literature; and (4) not identifying signs and symptoms of AMI by health care professionals. We used the exact search term in all the databases, search limits, inclusion, and exclusion criteria.

2.2.4 Methodology assessment

Two authors independently assessed the methodology of papers using the Newcastle-Ottawa Scales (NOS) for cross-sectional studies of research papers [25] which contains seven items categorized into three domains: (1) selection, (2) comparability, and (3) outcome. This scale is based on the star grading system, where the items can be rated from zero to two stars. The maximum achievable points are 10, which represents the highest methodological quality. The assessment of the methodological quality of the included papers was divided into three groups according to the overall assessment scores: low quality (0–4), moderate quality (5–6), and high quality (7–10) [26].

2.2.5 Data extraction and synthesis

A meta-analysis was inappropriate due to the samples' excessive heterogeneity and variation in the studies reviewed [27]; therefore, the findings are presented systematically. For each of the included studies, we extracted contextual information: author(s), year of publication, research design, the aim of the research, sample size, and funding source (Tab. 3.2). Data analysis was conducted through a thematic analysis of the included studies based on the recommendations by Thomas and Harden [28]. These guidelines for data analysis were chosen for their realistic approach, which tends to be more research-oriented and focus on contexts. Using these guidelines enabled the achievement of detailed data summaries from the included studies [29]. After reviewing the heterogeneity of the included studies, we extracted only primary and paraphrased statements of the results from each paper. Two authors independently read the extracted results of the included studies, defined the codes, and added the codes into the MaxQda program for further analysis and management of data. We undertook three steps to synthesize data: first, the authors searched through the texts and defined codes by reading each study line-by-line. Second, the authors identified codes from the first steps, refined them, and organized them into descriptive primary subthemes with an inductive approach. In the last step, we included the third author to review and discuss all the steps of thematic analysis, interpretation, and development of the descriptive primary level subthemes into secondary-level subthemes from which a thematic framework was developed.

2.3 Results

Using the search strategy and within the limits of the search, we found 1,434 records in CINAHL, 1,008 in MEDLINE, 4 in SAGE, and 368 in ScienceDirect. Additionally, we identified four through other sources. The records were imported into the EndNote program for managing references, and with the help of the program, we identified and removed duplicates. At first, two authors independently searched all titles and abstracts and chose those to be read in full based on the posed inclusion criteria studies. The steps of choosing the papers are displayed in Fig. 2.1.

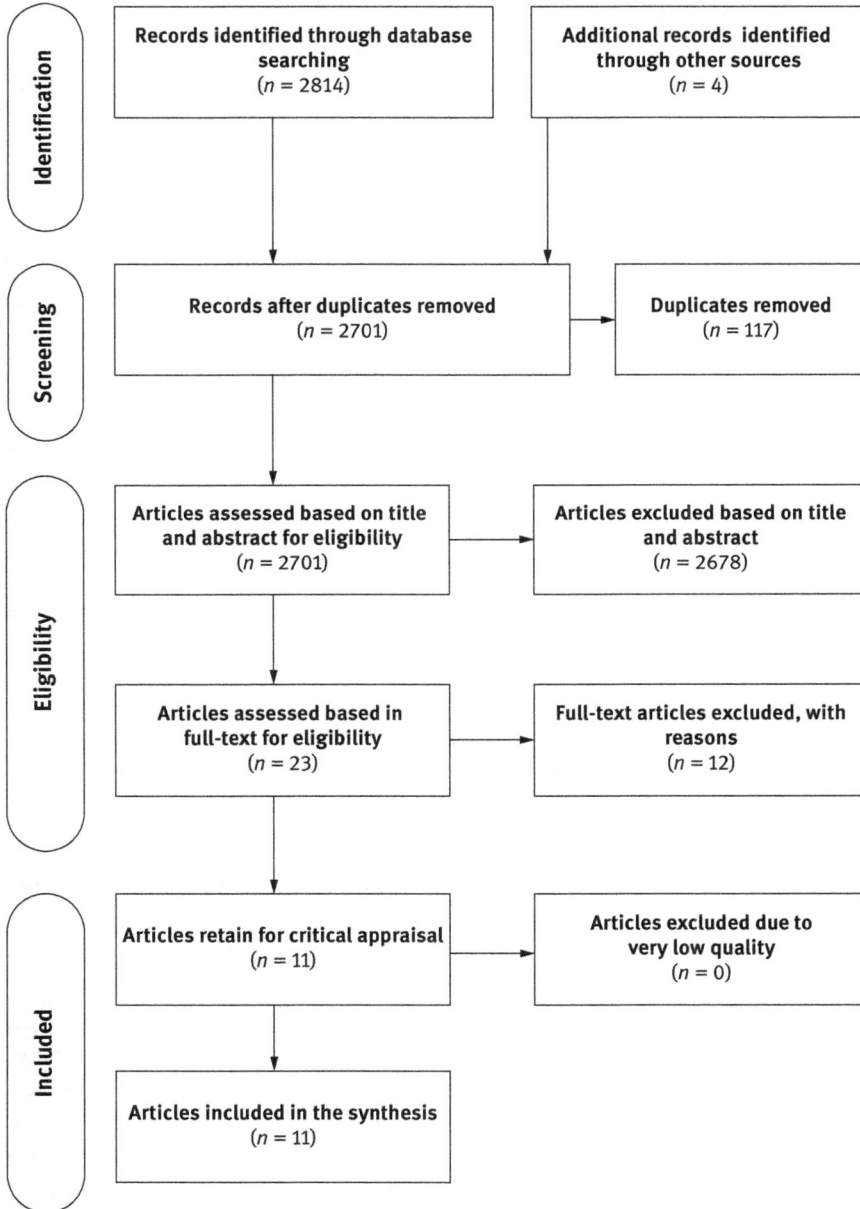

Fig. 2.1: The process of selecting the studies.

To achieve consistency and reduce bias, we included a third author. Cohen's kappa coefficient was used to assess the authors' agreement to increase the review's transparency and the risk of publishing. In the process of collecting (title, abstract, and full reading) the papers for review, the authors reached almost perfect agreement ($\kappa = 0.960$; $p = 0.001$), and similar results were obtained for determining risk of bias ($\kappa = 0.963$; $p = 0.001$). Of the 2,814 identified records, 11 papers matched the inclusion criteria and included detailed data extraction and analysis. The appraisal of the quality of evidence ranged from moderate to high. Most of the research papers (10/11) were high quality, and one study was deemed moderate (Tab. 2.1).

Tab. 2.1: Methodology assessment of each study.

Critically appraised papers	Selection (max. 5 stars)				Comparability (max. 2 stars)	Outcome (max. 3 stars)		Total scores
	1	2	3	4	5	6	7	
DeVon and Zerwic [30]	*	–	–	**	*	**	*	7
DeVon et al. [31]	*	*	*	**	*	**	*	9
McSweeney et al. [32]	*	*	*	**	*	**	*	9
Hwang et al. [33]	*	–	–	**	*	**	*	7
Morgan [34]	*	–	*	**	*	**	*	8
Løvlien et al. [35]	*	*	*	*	*	**	*	8
Kirchberger et al. [36]	*	*	*	–	*	**	*	7
Ahmed et al. [37]	*	–	*	**	*	**	*	8
Berg et al. [11]	*	–	*	**	*	**	*	7
DeVon et al. [8]	*	*	*	**	*	**	*	9
Kayhan et al. [38]	*	–	–	–	*	**	*	5

1, representativeness of the sample; 2, sample size; 3, non-respondents; 4, ascertainment of the exposure; 5, the subjects in different outcome groups are comparable, based on the study design or analysis; 6, assessment of the outcome; 7, statistical test; –, 0 point; *, 1 point; **,2 point; max., maximum.

We included 11 studies in a systematic review of the literature related to the detected symptoms in patients with myocardial infarction in the ED. No study used qualitative or mixed methods, and 11 used a quantitative design. The extraction of included studies is displayed in Tab. 2.2.

To identify detected symptoms and timespan for seeking help in patients with myocardial infarction, line-by-line coding for all studies enabled the identification of free codes ($n = 122$), leading to the development of six descriptive primary level subthemes: ACS; Associated disease; Women; Men; Older adults; and Younger adults. Through the analysis and comparison, we identified three secondary-level themes: illness, gender, and age. All themes were analysed to develop a thematic framework from which the one main theme was identified: Clinical symptoms. The results from the data synthesis of included studies can be found in Fig. 2.2.

Tab. 2.2: Characteristics of included papers.

Author; year; country	Research design	Aim of research	Sample size	Main findings related to detected symptoms
DeVon and Zerwic [30]; 2004; USA	Quantitative study; cross-sectional observational study	Discovering if symptoms of unstable angina pectoris (UAP) differed from acute myocardial infarction (AMI) symptoms	$n = 338$ ($n = 100$ patients with UAP and $n = 238$ patients with myocardial infarction)	– Patients with UAP more significantly reported dizziness ($p = 0.05$), numbness in the hands ($p < 0.01$), chest pain ($p = 0.05$), and unusual fear. – Patients with AMI more significantly reported nausea ($p = 0.05$), vomiting ($p < 0.001$), indigestion ($p < 0.01$), fatigue, and sweating. – Most patients experienced chest discomfort. – Patients with myocardial infarction evaluated chest pain higher ($\bar{x} = 8.46$; SD = 2.2), on the scale from 1 to 10, than patients with UAP ($\bar{x} = 7.69$; SD = 2.39; $t = 2.62$, $p < 0.01$).

(continued)

Tab. 2.2 (continued)

Author; year; country	Research design	Aim of research	Sample size	Main findings related to detected symptoms
DeVon and Ryan [31]; 2008; US A	Quantitative study; cross-sectional observational study	To indicate symptoms difference between women and men with unstable angina pectoris, myocardial infarction without ST elevation, and myocardial infarction with ST-elevation. They follow age, anxiety, depression, functional status, and diabetes	$n = 256$ ($n = 112$ women and $n = 144$ men)	– More than half of all patients answered that their symptoms were not caused by effort, emotional agitation, or rest. – Women complained more often about indigestion ($p = 0.04$), palpitation ($p = 0.02$), nausea ($p < 0.01$), numbness in the hands ($p = 0.03$), and unusual fatigue ($p < 0.01$). – Women more often reported pain in the jaw ($p = 0.02$) and in the neck ($p < 0.01$) compared to men. – Men with elevated ST myocardial infarction more often complained about dizziness ($p < 0.01$). – Women with unstable angina pectoris and without elevated ST myocardial infarction felt weakness more often ($p < 0.01$). – Women with elevated ST AMI complained of newly existing cough more often ($p < 0.01$). – Women described chest pain as feeling anxious ($p = 0.03$) and tingling; on the other hand, men described their pain as burning.

McSweeney et al. [32]; 2010; US A	Quantitative study; multicentre retrospective research	To compare cardiovascular disease warning signs with AIM symptoms in women of black, Latin, and white races	$n = 1,270$ ($n = 454$ black women, $n = 539$ white women and $n = 186$ Latino women)	– 95% of all women, regardless of race, reported early prodromal symptoms, and the most common symptom was fatigue.
				– Anxiety was the second most common symptom in Latino women ($p < 0.001$).
				– Chest pain/discomfort was the most common symptom in Latino and white women and the second most common symptom in black women.
				– Black women reported two generalized symptoms: feeling hot and indigestion more often than Latino and white women ($p < 0.001$).
Hwang et al. [33]; 2006; US A	Quantitative methodology; cross-sectional observational study	Investigate the effect of age on the onset of symptoms	$n = 239$ (older adults older more than 65 years old ($n = 96$) and younger adults younger than $n = 143$ 65 years old)	– Older adults (65–89 years old) more often had hypertension ($p < 0.001$), diabetes, and a history of stroke ($p = 0.05$).
				– Older adults had significantly fewer symptoms than younger adults; symptoms that appear more often are weakness, sweating, fear, nausea, and indigestion ($p = 0.05$).
				– 58% of older adults said that experienced symptoms were not the same as expected.

(continued)

Tab. 2.2 (continued)

Author; year; country	Research design	Aim of research	Sample size	Main findings related to detected symptoms
Morgan [34]; 2005; USA	Quantitative study; correlation study	The aim was to determine the extent of incompatibility between AMI's expected and actual symptoms	n = 110 (62 men and 36 women)	– Women reported pain in hands, arms, jaw, and neck more often than men. – Men more often reported symptoms like dizziness, nausea, headache, sweating, and shortness of breath. – In women, fatigue (p = 0.05), nausea and vomiting, dizziness, and numbness in hands or palms were dominant symptoms. – Heartburn or indigestion, diarrhoea, and dizziness appeared approximately the same in both sexes. – The most common symptom that patients expected was chest pain; that same symptom was the most common.
Løvlien et al. [35]; 2006; Norway	Quantitative methodology; cross-sectional retrospective study	Compare the symptoms and course of the disease in both genders with diagnosed AIM	n = 82 (patients aged up to 65 years old who had their first AIM)	– Chest pain was the most common symptom in both genders. – Women and men who were 50 years old or less often experienced pain in both arms (p < 0.01). Men and women older than 50 reported back pain (p = 0.05). – More men (84%) than women (66%) attributed the pain to heart disease (p = 0.05). – Women who did not attribute their symptoms to heart disease had chest pain and arm pain (33%).

Kirchberger et al. [36]; 2016; Germany	Quantitative study; observational retrospective study	Consider the frequency of symptom mismatching and which factors are associated with the mismatching of symptoms	n = 1,282 (n = 990 men and n = 292 women)	– Among all patients, 94.3% had a different range of expressed symptoms at re-infarction compared to the first infraction.
				– According to a re-infarction, men have a lower probability of mismatching symptoms at first infarction in pain between shoulder blades and jaw/neck, nausea, vomit, and fear of death than women.
				– Several mismatching symptoms at first infarction and re-infarction were significantly lower in men than in women (p < 0.001).
Ahmed et al. [37]; 2018; Pakistan	Quantitative methodology; cross-sectional study	Evaluate the symptoms in patients with myocardial infarction and diabetes or without diabetes	n = 280 (n = 130 patients with diabetes and n = 150 non-diabetes patients)	– Chest pain was the most common symptom in patients with diabetes and those without diabetes.
				– Patients with diabetes reported less often chest pain than patients without diabetes (77.7% vs 86.7%) (p = 0.049).
				– Sweating, dyspnoea, nausea, and vomiting are symptoms that have appeared equally common in patients with and without diabetes.

(continued)

Tab. 2.2 (continued)

Author; year; country	Research design	Aim of research	Sample size	Main findings related to detected symptoms
Berg et al. [11]; 2009; Sweden	Quantitative methodology; retrospective study	Analyses the differences in experiencing symptoms of AMI between gender	$n = 225$ ($n = 52$ women and $n = 173$ men)	– Most women and men had pain in the chest. There was no significant difference between gender. – Nausea has been more often in women (53.8%) than in men (29.5%). – Women reported pain in the back (odds ratio – OR = 4.29) and dizziness (OR = 2.60). – Women had a higher number of symptoms (4–6) than men (3) ($p = 0.04$). – Central (squeezing) chest pain is the most common pain in both genders.
DeVon et al. [8]; 2014; USA	Quantitative study; prospective study	To investigate differences in symptoms between black and white patients who arrived at an emergency	$n = 663$ ($n = 116$ black patients and $n = 547$ white patients)	– Black patients report more symptoms than white patients. – Black patients complain more often about pressure and pain in the chest, sweating ($p < 0.001$), pain in the upper back ($p < 0.001$), and palpitation ($p = 0.05$) than white patients.
Kayhan et al. [38]; 2017; Turkey	Quantitative study; retrospective study	The aim was to identify symptoms in patients diagnosed with AMI admitted to the ED	$n = 285$ ($n = 59$ women and $n = 226$ men)	– The most common symptom in men and women with STEMI and NSTEMI is chest pain. – Patients with NSTEMI more often complain about pain in the left arm and dyspnoea than patients with STEMI.

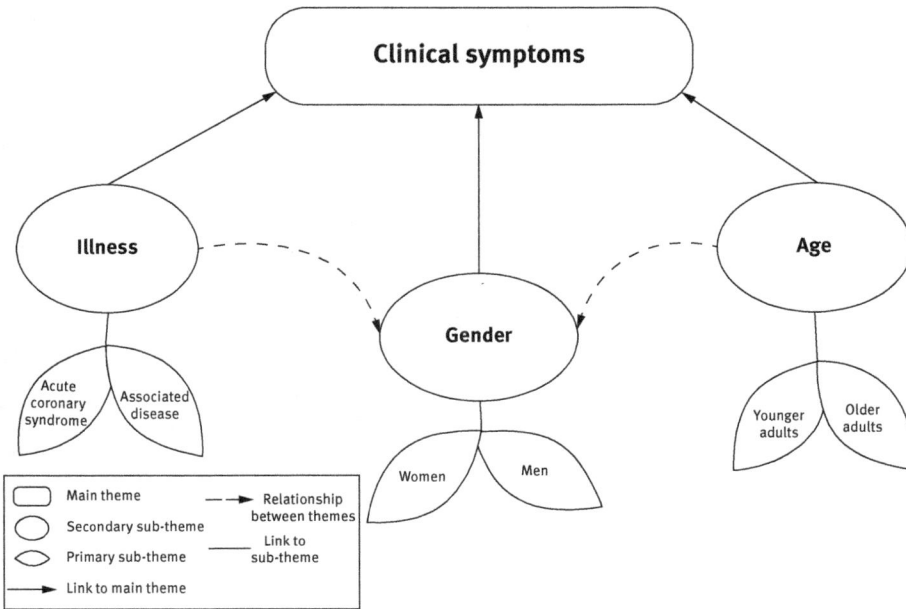

Fig. 2.2: The results from data synthesis of included studies.

2.3.1 Clinical symptoms

Three secondary-level subthemes were defined within clinical symptoms: illness, gender, and age.

Illness

The subtheme of illness contains two descriptive elements: ACS and associated diseases. Certain differences in the occurrence of symptoms regarding the type of AMI have been identified [37]. Among patients with myocardial infarction, those diagnosed with STEMI (77.5%) dominate compared to NSTEMI (22.5%) [38]. The most commonly expressed symptom, regardless of the type of AMI, is chest pain [27, 37], which appeared in all identified studies. Ahmed et al. [37] note that chest pain is the most common symptom identified by patients with diabetes and those without it. Furthermore, they note that patients with diabetes are less likely to report chest pain (77.5%) as compared with patients without diabetes (86.7%) ($p = 0.049$). Patients with NSTEMI more frequently report dyspnoea and pain in their left shoulder (7.81%); meanwhile, patients with STEMI more frequently report nausea (3.16%)

and syncope (3.62%). However, regardless of the type of AMI, there is no statistically significant difference in those symptoms ($p = 0.458$) [38].

Gender

A secondary subtheme of gender includes two descriptive primary subthemes. Chest pain is the most common symptom, regardless of gender [11, 31, 32, 34, 35, 38]. In symptoms like pain in the hands or arms, sweating, dyspnoea, tiredness, neck and back pain, abdominal or epigastric pain, vomiting, syncope, nausea, heartburn, diarrhoea, and jaw pain, a significant statistical difference was not found between genders ($p = 0.260$) [11, 38]. The average number of symptoms patients had was slightly higher in women than in men, but there was a small difference [31]. Berg et al. [11] similarly note that women, on average, report a more significant number of symptoms (between 4 and 6) than men, who report, on average, three symptoms ($p = 0.04$) [36].

Age

Hwang et al. [33] note that older adults (65–89 years old) more frequently had associated diseases like arterial hypertension ($p < 0.001$), diabetes mellitus, and a history of stroke ($p = 0.05$). Older adults also significantly less frequently reported pain in the middle of their chest area ($p = 0.05$) and less frequently complained about sweating, fear, indigestion ($p = 0.05$), nausea, fainting, and dizziness, which dominated in younger adults (31–64 years old). Expressed pain intensity is not significantly different between young and older adult patients. Young adults more frequently reported pain as burning ($p = 0.05$), sharp ($p = 0.05$), and heavy ($p = 0.05$) in comparison with older adults. The appearance of shortness of breath, tiredness, weakness, vomiting, and palpitation is not significantly different with regard to the age of the patients. Older adults complained about fewer symptoms in comparison with younger adults. Fifty-eight per cent of older adult patients reported that the expected symptoms of AMI were not the same as they experienced [33].

2.4 Discussion

Based on our systematic review of the literature on the perceived symptoms of AMI that help triage nurses to identify timely, we identified that the most common symptom, regardless of the kind of AMI or gender, is chest pain [11, 30–32, 34, 39]. Other symptoms include nausea, vomiting [30], and indigestion [31, 32]. Shortness of breath, tiredness, weakness [31, 32, 34], sweating, neck, and jaw pain [11] can also appear. Kayhan et al. [38] identified that patients report shortness of breath, tiredness, weakness, and sweating to roughly the same extent, regardless of whether diagnosed with UAP or AMI. Further, McSweeney et al. [32], Morgan [34], DeVon et al. [31] and Ryan et al. [19] report that the most common symptoms of AMI in females, regardless of race, are shortness of breath, weakness, and fatigue. Berg, Björck [11] also note that sweating, tiredness, neck and jaw pain, dyspnoea, abdominal pain, and syncope appear in both men and women with the same frequency. Kayhan et al. [38] similarly report incidences of dyspnoea and syncope between the sexes, as with pain in the left shoulder and back.

Our review identified that patients with AMI commonly report nausea and vomiting [30, 38], which is more common among women [34]. Additional research [31, 35, 38] found similar results for nausea alone. Kayhan et al. [38] state that the appearance of nausea and vomiting in men and women does not significantly differ.

Men reported worse pain than women and further reported similar locations and the quality of the pain [31]. Berg et al. [11] describe that women had occasional pain that was not long-lasting. According to Hwang et al. [33], young adults more frequently reported pain in the middle of their chest in comparison with the older adults. Older adults described the pain as burning, sharp, and challenging [33].

In the ED, the diagnosis needs to be initiated when the patient arrives, and the main complaints present as typical or atypical symptoms of AMI to the triage nurse. Jaeger, Wildi [39] state that it may be possible to diagnose AMI with the help of anamnesis, physical examination, 12-lead ECG, pulse oximetry, standard laboratory test, and chest radiography. Furthermore, Body et al. [40] recommended additional tests such as measuring a high-sensitivity cardiac troponin concentration, age, risk factors, and Troponin (HEART) score or the Troponin-only Manchester Acute Coronary Syndromes (T-MACS) decision aid. With these specific algorithms, we can calculate each individual patient's probability of AMI following a single blood test at the time of arrival at the ED to guide decision-making [41]. Furthermore, T-MACS identify individuals at high risk of AMI who require referral to cardiology [42].

2.4.1 Recommendations

Our chapter presents the symptoms and signs triage nurses detect in AMI patients seeking help at an ED. More research is necessary that focuses on timely identification of symptoms that indicate AMI, the role of decision-making skills in determining the appropriate triage category for those patients and follow-up action by healthcare practitioners in EDs. Furthermore, emphasis should be placed on researching the influence of education, knowledge, resources, and skills among triage nurses in relation to the timely identification of symptoms of AMI as a life-threatening condition.

2.4.2 Limitations

This review has several limitations. Some important papers have probably been excluded based on the eligibility criteria. Also, this review included only studies published in English, and this criterion may have excluded relevant literature published in other languages as the translation was unavailable. Quality assessment was performed with the NOS, which is a useful tool, although its reliability could be improved by an additional assessment of the methodological quality of the included studies. To reduce reporting bias, we followed the recommendations by Higgins and Green [29] and the PRISMA Checklist [24].

2.5 Conclusion

Based on a literature review, the most frequently detected symptom in AMI patients is chest pain. In patients with AMI, various symptoms range from typical chest pain, shortness of breath, sweating, and pain in the hands, to atypical symptoms such as indigestion, weakness, numbness in the hands, and upper abdominal pain, anxiety, and headache. We found that men are more likely to report abdominal pain, left shoulder pain, headache, dizziness, and nausea than women, who often experience fatigue, vomiting, nausea, and collapse. Race, gender, age, and associated diseases, especially diabetes mellitus, affect the onset of symptoms. Furthermore, we discovered that women report more symptoms (from 4 to 6), while men, on average, report three symptoms. Thus, triage nurses need to pay attention to cardiovascular symptoms. Their focus also needs to be redirected to epigastric pain and cold sweating, which are abdominal and systemic symptoms, and anxiety and nausea/vomiting in patients with diabetes.

References

[1] Thomas H, Diamond J, Vieco A, Chaudhuri S, Shinnar E, Cromer S, et al. Global atlas of cardiovascular disease. Glob Heart, 2018, 13, 143–163.
[2] Rashidi A, Whitehead L, Glass C. Factors affecting hospital readmission rates following an acute coronary syndrome: A systematic review. J Clin Nurs, 2021.
[3] Holc I. Akutni koronarni sindrom. In: Holc I, Križmarić M, Mekiš D, Pajnkihar M, Kamenik M, Eds. Klinična patofiziologija nujnih stanj: Izbrana poglavja. Maribor, Univerza v Mariboru, Fakulteta za zdravstvene vede, 2016, 145–151.
[4] Štajer D, Koželj M. Kardiologija. In: Košnik M, Mrevlje F, Štajer D, et al., Eds. Interna medicina. 4th ed. Ljubljana, Littera picta, Slovensko medicinsko društvo, 2011, 113–351.
[5] Bevc S, Penko M, Zorman T. Simulacija akutnega koronarnega sindroma pri predmetu Interna medicina: Učno gradivo. 6. izd. ed. Maribor, Medicinska fakulteta, 2015, 21 f. p.

[6]   Bandstein N, Ljung R, Johansson M, Holzmann MJ. Undetectable high-sensitivity cardiac troponin T level in the ED and risk of myocardial infarction. J Am Coll Cardiol, 2014, 63(23), 2569–2578.

[7]   Banharak S, Prasankok C, Lach HW. Factors related to a delay in seeking treatment for acute myocardial infarction in older adults: An integrative review. Pac Rim Int J Nurs Res, 2020, 24(4), 553–568.

[8]   DeVon HA, Burke LA, Nelson H, Zerwic JJ, Riley B. Disparities in patients presenting to the ED with potential acute coronary syndrome: It matters if you are Black or White. Heart & Lung, 2014, 43(4), 270–277.

[9]   Fu R, Li S-D, Song C-X, Yang J-A, Xu H-Y, Gao X-J, et al. Clinical significance of diabetes on symptom and patient delay among patients with acute myocardial infarction – an analysis from China Acute Myocardial Infarction (CAMI) registry. J Geriatr Cardiol, 2019, 16(5), 395.

[10]   Lichtman JH, Leifheit EC, Safdar B, Bao H, Krumholz HM, Lorenze NP, et al. Sex differences in the presentation and perception of symptoms among young patients with myocardial infarction: Evidence from the VIRGO study (variation in recovery: Role of gender on outcomes of young AMI patients). Circulation, 2018, 137(8), 781–790.

[11]   Berg J, Björck L, Dudas K, Lappas G, Rosengren A. Symptoms of a first acute myocardial infarction in women and men. Gender Med, 2009, 6(3), 454–462.

[12]   Thygesen K, Alpert JS, Jaffe AS, Simoons ML, Chaitman BR, White HD, et al. Third universal definition of myocardial infarction. J Am Coll Cardiol, 2012, 60(16), 1581–1598.

[13]   Soares Passinho R, Garcia Romero Sipolatti W, Fioresi M, Caniçali Primo C. Signs, symptoms and complications of acute myocardial infarction. Rev Enferm, 2018, 12(1), 247–264.

[14]   Ekwall A, Gerdtz M, Manias E. The influence of patient acuity on satisfaction with emergency care: Perspectives of family, friends and carers. J Clin Nurs, 2008, 17(6), 800–809.

[15]   Fekonja Z, Pajnkihar M. Implementation of Manchester triage system in an ED in Slovenia. Egészség-akadémia, 2016, 7(3), 151–158.

[16]   Forsman B, Forsgren S, Carlström ED. Nurses working with Manchester triage–the impact of experience on patient security. Aust Emerg Nurs J, 2012, 15(2), 100–107.

[17]   Shamsi NM. Improving vital signs measurement and documentation in the triage room: A quality improvement project. Bahrain Med Bull, 2018, 40(3), 171–173.

[18]   Arslanian-Engoren C. Explicating nurses' cardiac triage decisions. J Cardiovasc Nurs, 2009, 24(1), 50–57.

[19]   Ryan K, Greenslade J, Dalton E, Chu K, Brown AF, Cullen L. Factors associated with triage assignment of ED patients ultimately diagnosed with acute myocardial infarction. Aust Crit Care, 2016, 29(1), 23–26.

[20]   Andersson H, Ullgren A, Holmberg M, Karlsson T, Herlitz J, Wireklint Sundström B. Acute coronary syndrome in relation to the occurrence of associated symptoms: A quantitative study in prehospital emergency care. Int Emerg Nurs, 2016, 33.

[21]   Canto AJ, Kiefe CI, Goldberg RJ, Rogers WJ, Peterson ED, Wenger NK, et al. Differences in symptom presentation and hospital mortality according to type of acute myocardial infarction. Am Heart J, 2012, 163(4), 572–579.

[22]   Reblora JM, Lopez V, Goh Y-S. Experiences of nurses working in a triage area: An integrative review. Aust Crit Care, 2020, 33(6), 567–575.

[23]   Hollander JE, Than M, Mueller C. State-of-the-art evaluation of ED patients presenting with potential acute coronary syndromes. Circulation, 2016, 134(7), 547–564.

[24]   Moher D, Liberati A, Tetzlaff J, Altman DG, The PG. Preferred reporting items for systematic reviews and meta-analyses: The PRISMA statement. PLOS Med, 2009, 6(7), e1000097.

[25] Modesti PA, Reboldi G, Cappuccio FP, Agyemang C, Remuzzi G, Rapi S, et al. Panethnic differences in blood pressure in Europe: A systematic review and meta-analysis. PloS One, 2016, 11(1), e0147601.

[26] Bowatte G, Tham R, Allen K, Tan D, Lau M, Dai X, et al. Breastfeeding and childhood acute otitis media: A systematic review and meta-analysis. Acta Paediatr, 2015, 104, 85–95.

[27] Kastrin A. Metaanaliza in njen pomen za psihološko metodologijo. Psihološka Obzorja, 2008, 17(3), 25–42.

[28] Thomas J, Harden A. Methods for the thematic synthesis of qualitative research in systematic reviews. BMC Med Res Methodol, 2008, 8(1), 1–10.

[29] Higgins J, Green S. Cochrane handbook for systematic review so interventions (version 5.0.2): The Cochrane Collaboration 2009. (Available from: http://handbook.cochrane.org).

[30] DeVon HA, Zerwic JJ. Differences in the symptoms associated with unstable angina and myocardial infarction. Prog Cardiovasc Dis Nurs, 2004, 19(1), 6–11.

[31] DeVon HA, Ryan CJ, Ochs AL, Shapiro M. Symptoms across the continuum of acute coronary syndromes: Differences between women and men. Am J Crit Care, 2008, 17(1), 14–24, quiz 5.

[32] McSweeney JC, O'Sullivan P, Cleves MA, Lefler LL, Cody M, Moser DK, et al. Racial differences in women's prodromal and acute symptoms of myocardial infarction. Am J Crit Care, 2010, 19(1), 63–73.

[33] Hwang SY, Ryan C, Zerwic JJ. The influence of age on acute myocardial infarction symptoms and patient delay in seeking treatment. Prog Cardiovasc Dis Nurs, 2006, 21(1), 20–27.

[34] Morgan DM. Effect of incongruence of acute myocardial infarction symptoms on the decision to seek treatment in a rural population. J Cardiovasc Nurs, 2005, 20(5), 365–371.

[35] Løvlien M, Schei B, Gjengedal E. Are there gender differences related to symptoms of acute myocardial infarction? A Norwegian perspective. Prog Cardiovasc Dis Nurs, 2006, 21(1), 14–19.

[36] Kirchberger I, Heier M, Golüke H, Kuch B, von Scheidt W, Peters A, et al. Mismatch of presenting symptoms at first and recurrent acute myocardial infarction. From the MONICA/KORA Myocardial Infarction Registry. Eur J Prev Cardiol, 2016, 23(4), 377–384.

[37] Ahmed S, Khan A, Ali SI, Saad M, Jawaid H, Islam M, et al. Differences in symptoms and presentation delay times in myocardial infarction patients with and without diabetes: A cross-sectional study in Pakistan. Indian Heart J, 2018, 70(2), 241–245.

[38] Kayhan M, Mamur A, Ünlüoğlu İ, Balcıoğlu H, Acar N, Bilge U. An assessment of initial symptoms in patients admitted to the ER of a tertiary healthcare institution and diagnosed with acute myocardial infarction. Biomed Res Ther, 2017, 28(9), 4202–4207.

[39] Jaeger C, Wildi K, Twerenbold R, Reichlin T, Gimenez MR, Neuhaus J-D, et al. One-hour rule-in and rule-out of acute myocardial infarction using high-sensitivity cardiac troponin I. Am Heart J, 2016, 171(1), 92–102.

[40] Body R, Almashali M, Morris N, Moss P, Jarman H, Appelboam A, et al. Diagnostic accuracy of the T-MACS decision aid with a contemporary point-of-care troponin assay. Heart, 2019, 105(10), 768–774.

[41] Body R. Acute coronary syndromes diagnosis, version 2.0: Tomorrow's approach to diagnosing acute coronary syndromes?. Turk J Emerg Med, 2018, 18(3), 94–99.

[42] Greenslade JH, Carlton EW, Van Hise C, Cho E, Hawkins T, Parsonage WA, et al. Diagnostic accuracy of a new high-sensitivity troponin I assay and five accelerated diagnostic pathways for ruling out acute myocardial infarction and acute coronary syndrome. Ann Emerg Med, 2018, 71(4), 439–451. e3.

Leona Cilar Budler, Sergej Kmetec, Gregor Štiglic,
Kathy Leadbitter, Sabina Herle, Klavdija Čuček Trifkovič

3 Mental well-being of parents of children with autism spectrum disorder in Slovenia

Abstract

Introduction: Autism spectrum disorder refers to neurodevelopmental disabilities that affect social, communicative, and behavioural development. Parents of children with autism spectrum disorder often face parenting challenges, such as difficulties understanding and communicating with their children. Such factors can lead to poor mental well-being. Mental well-being is a state of positive psychological and emotional health.

Methods: A cross-sectional study was conducted to determine whether there was a relationship between parental mental well-being and family experience. The Autism Family Experience Questionnaire measured family experience and quality of life. The Warwick Edinburgh Mental Well-being Scale measured parents' mental well-being.

Results: A total of 101 parents of children with autism spectrum disorder from Slovenia participated in the study. A small correlation between parental mental well-being and the positive family experience was found. The mental well-being of parents negatively correlates with family life and child symptoms and positively with the experience of being a parent and child development. Parents reported poor support from the health system. Parents who devote more time to themselves also have better mental well-being. Parents report a lack of support from health professionals, resulting in poor mental well-being.

Discussion and conclusion: An integrated person-centred approach should be introduced to reduce stress, emotional burden, and physical fatigue by the parents of children with autism spectrum disorder and improve their mental well-being. Future research could investigate possible solutions for improving the mental well-being of parents of children with autism spectrum disorder.

Keywords: Autism spectrum disorder, mental well-being, child, parenting, cross-sectional studies

3.1 Introduction

Autism spectrum disorder (ASD) is a complex neurodevelopmental condition characterized by persistent communication and social interaction impairment and restricted and repetitive activities, behaviour, and interests [1]. Parenting a child with ASD can present a daily challenge for parents and can significantly affect their mental well-being [2, 3], quality of life [4, 5], and family life [6]. Furthermore, parents of children with ASD often experience increased stress, symptoms of depression, or other psychological problems [7–9]. Elevated stress levels may occur when parents' demand exceed their coping resources [2].

Mental well-being is a positive state of psychological and emotional health [10]. It varies among the different sociocultural contexts of each individual [11]. Numerous factors can affect the well-being of parents of children with ASD. Authors argued that behavioural problems are the most important predictors of parental stress in children with ASD and other disabilities [12]. Other key factors include the child's age [13], regulatory problems, and increased autism severity [12]. Parents with increased self-blame because of their child's health condition or despair have poorer mental well-being [14]. Other factors that may impact parents' mental well-being are inadequate access to mental health services [15], poor physical health [16], and lower quality of life [17]. Contextual factors contributing to stress include financial strain [18], misunderstanding of child's condition, judgement and stigma related to child's condition [12], a lack of cooperation between parents and healthcare workers [19], lack of understanding and support from family, and even from some professionals [12].

There is very little research into the experiences of parents and families of children with ASD in Slovenia. Support services may not be as well developed in Slovenia as in other countries in Europe or the United States of America (USA). A 2017 Slovene study by Schmidt et al. [20] highlighted the need for appropriate and efficient support for families with children with ASD. Slovenian parents stated in an online blog that no comprehensive treatment is available within the healthcare system and that appropriate treatment is not accessible to all parents [21]. There is a gap in understanding Slovene families' needs, that is, how parents experience parenting a child with ASD and its effect on their mental well-being. The chapter aims to explore whether there are differences in ASD family experiences or parental mental well-being related to different demographic factors and find out if there is an association between parent mental well-being and family experience with ASD.

3.2 Methods

A cross-sectional study was conducted to determine whether there was a relationship between parental mental well-being and family experience with ASD.

3.2.1 Participants

Participants were recruited over 60 days (March–May 2018) via e-mail addresses obtained from non-governmental services (NGOs) and social media invitations. A total of 101 parents of children with ASD participated in the study: 86 (85.1%) were mothers and 15 (14.9%) were fathers (Tab. 3.1).

Tab. 3.1: Sample characteristics.

Variables	*n*	%
Gender		
Male	15	14.9
Female	86	85.1
Employment		
Yes	79	78.2
No	22	21.8
Highest educational level		
Unfinished elementary school	1	1.0
Secondary school	28	27.7
Higher education program	16	15.8
University-level programs (first degree)	21	20.8
Master level (second degree)	34	33.6
PhD level (third degree)	1	1.1

n, number of participants; %, per cent.

3.2.2 Measures

The Autism Family Experience Questionnaire (AFEQ) is a scale developed in the UK to measure family experience, quality of life, and prioritized outcomes for early intervention in families of children with ASD [22]. The questionnaire is divided into four subdomains. The first domain (experience being a parent of a child with autism) relates to parental battles and realistic expectations about the child's development. The second domain (family life) was developed based on wider family attitudes, routines, and structures at home. The third domain (child development) refers to the child's development, understanding, and social relationships. The fourth domain (child symptoms) refers to the feelings and behaviour of the child. Data from the AFEQ within non-United Kingdom (UK) cultural contexts have not been published.

The AFEQ questionnaire was translated to Slovenian following a standardized procedure [23]. First, two independent bilingual translators performed a translation of the questionnaire from the original English into the Slovenian language. The first translator (LCB) was aware of the concepts in the questionnaire and aimed to provide a translation in which meanings were consistent with the original instrument. The second translator (SK) was not unaware of the questionnaire's objective. Disagreements were discussed with a third researcher (GS). Second, the translated version of the questionnaire was back-translated into English. Differences with the original version were discussed with the questionnaire author (KL) and adjusted accordingly to ensure that the original meaning was maintained.

The Warwick-Edinburgh Mental Well-being Scale (WEMWBS) is a scale developed in the UK in 2006. It is a 14-item, 5-level scale ranging from "none of the time" to "all the time". It measures all attributes of mental well-being, except spirituality [24].

A bespoke questionnaire consisted of 14 questions: parentage; gender; employment; education level; region; number of children in the family and number of children with ASD; age of the child with ASD; hours devoted to care of the child with ASD and to themselves; satisfaction with life; satisfaction with healthcare support; help with child with ASD; involvement in school; and support from NGOs.

3.2.3 Data analysis

Data were analysed using descriptive and inferential statistics in R statistical computing environment [25]. AFEQ items that were negatively worded were scored in reverse order, consistent with the scoring guidelines. A minimum possible score of AFEQ was 48 and a maximum of 240, where lower scores represent better experience. A minimum score of WEMWBS was 14 and a maximum of 70, where higher scores represent better mental well-being. All items were worded positively in WEMWBS. The total score for both scales was calculated by totalling the scores for each item with equal weights. No missing data were recorded. Since none of the tested sub-groups deviated from the normal distribution, we used Pearson correlation coefficient (r_p) to measure correlation, a t-test of independent samples when comparing the mean values of two groups, and an ANOVA analysis of variance analyses the differences among group means. When comparing the AFEQ mean to the original study from the UK, a one-sample t-test was used.

3.3 Results

3.3.1 Descriptive data and internal consistency

A summary of variables related to family and satisfaction with life is presented in Tab. 3.2.

Tab. 3.2: Summary of variables related to family, time devoted to child and self, and satisfaction-related questions.

Variables	*n*	%
Number of children in the family		
One	33	32.7
Two	45	44.6
Three	15	14.9
Four or more	8	7.8
Hours devoted to the care of a child with ASD (per day)		
1–6	69	68.4
7–12	19	18.8
13–18	2	2.0
19–24	11	10.8
Hours devoted to self-care (per day)		
Zero	34	33.7
One	42	41.6
Two	18	17.7
Three or more	7	7.0
General satisfaction with life		
Yes	43	42.6
No	34	33.7
I do not know	21	20.7
I do not want to answer	3	3.0
Satisfaction with healthcare support		
Satisfied	5	5.0
Unsatisfied	90	89.1
Do not know	6	5.9

n, number of participants; %, per cent.

The minimum score on the AFEQ was 123, and the maximum was 158, with a mean of 138.3 (SD = 7.9). The mean of the AFEQ in this study was lower (i.e., better) than baseline scores in the original [22] study and slightly higher compared the follow-up period to original study at (M = 141.0, SD = 21.3, p < 0.001; M = 133.0, SD = 22.8, p < 0.001).

Nevertheless, the minimum value was 123 when the original study minimum was 81.8 (78.1 at follow-up), suggesting a smaller range of experience in the Slovenian sample. Cronbach's α for AFEQ total score was 0.648. The relatively low alpha value in AFEQ may be due to poor interrelatedness between items or heterogeneous constructs.

A minimum score of WEMWBS was 24 and a maximum of 67, with a mean of 46.3 (SD = 8.8). According to the National Health Service (NHS) [26] classification, the mean score of the mental well-being of parents in this sample was average. Cronbach's α for WEMWBS was 0.918. A high alpha value in WEMWBS shows that items correlate and have a high degree of internal consistency.

3.3.2 Relationship between autism family experience, parental mental well-being, and demographic factors

There was a very small and non-significant difference ($t(99) = 1.036$, $p = 0.303$) in family experience with autism scores of fathers ($M = 140.3$, SD = 7.4) compared with mothers ($M = 138.0$, SD = 7.9). Family experience with ASD differed according to the employment status of the parents ($t(99) = -2.412$, $p = 0.018$), where employed parents achieved a mean score of 137.4 (SD = 7.5) and unemployed parents achieved a score of 141.8 (SD = 8.3). The correlation between family experience with autism and levels of education was not significant ($r_p = -0.093$, $n = 101$, $p = 0.355$). We were also not able to confirm significant differences in family experience among parents with different number of children ($F(5, 95) = 2.139$, $p = 0.067$). Parents who devote more time to themselves scored higher in WEMWBS score, suggesting better mental well-being ($r_p = 0.224$, $n = 101$, $p = 0.025$). The correlation between WEMWBS score and time devoted to children was small and non-significant ($r_p = -0.106$, $n = 101$, $p = 0.294$).

3.3.3 Correlation between family experience with autism and parents' mental well-being

The correlation between mental well-being and family experience with autism was analysed using Pearson correlation coefficient. There was a significant negative correlation (better autism family experience correlates with higher well-being) between the two variables ($r_p = -0.312$, $n = 101$, $p < 0.001$). According to the strength levels of the correlation by Evans [27], the correlation between the two variables is small. Furthermore, subdomains of the AFEQ were also tested for correlation with WEMWBS (Tab. 3.3).

The mental well-being of parents negatively correlates with family life and child symptoms and positively with the experience of being a parent and child development.

Tab. 3.3: Correlation of autism family experience and mental well-being.

		WEMWBS	
		r_p	p
AFEQ	**Family life**	−0.502	< 0.001*
	Experience of being a parent	0.375	< 0.001*
	Child development	0.001	0.994
	Child symptoms	−0.306	0.002*
	AFEQ total	−0.312	0.001*

AFEQ, The Autism Family Experience Questionnaire; p, statistical significance; r_p, Pearson correlation coefficient; WEMWBS, The Warwick-Edinburgh Mental Well-being Scale; *, statistical significance p-value (≤ 0.05).

3.4 Discussion

The mean AFEQ score in our study was approximately three points lower (better), and there was a smaller variation in scores (SD of 7.9 compared to 21.3) compared with the baseline scores of the original study [22]. In interpreting these results, the authors must consider the differences between the participants in the UK study [22] and ours. Furthermore, this leads to a more heterogeneous response from the UK parents than in the Slovenian sample. This may be because the UK sample was young and recently diagnosed. Therefore, parents may still have been in a period of adaptation and adjustment to their child's diagnosis leading to more variability in their reports of their family experience and quality of life. Many participants in the Slovenian sample were recruited through an NGO that supports autistic people and their parents. They might have received more support regarding their child with ASD than is typical in Slovenia, which could explain the slightly higher scores on the questionnaire.

The mean score of mental well-being for this sample (M = 46.3; SD = 8.8) would be classified as average and slightly lower than the results (M = 47.8; SD = 4.7) in a general population of parents [28]. It is perhaps surprising that the mean mental well-being score within this sample of parents of children with ASD is in the "average" range. Therefore, this seems to contradict previous findings that family members of a child with ASD experience poorer mental well-being and increased stress [29–31]. However, our study's median of the WEMWBS is 45, which is lower (M = 51.0). It also seems to run contrary to the fact that 89% of the sample are dissatisfied with health-care support. The WEMWBS tool is limited only to current mental well-being, which might not correlate with long-term dissatisfaction. Further research could explore this finding further in other samples within Slovenia and similar countries.

Several factors were not associated with AFEQ scores: parent gender; education level; or several children in the family. Parental mental well-being was associated with employment status (with better family experience reported by parents in employment) and the amount of time devoted to themselves. These findings emphasize the importance of contextual factors to well-being in families of children with ASD. Employment can bring financial stability and the opportunity for parents to experience life outside the home. Time to oneself may be particularly important when raising a child with ASD and may provide opportunities to rest, exercise, and enjoy hobbies or other activities that improve well-being. Parents with more time to themselves may have increased social support, and better social support has contributed to better parental mental well-being [32]. The AFEQ is developed to measure family experience, quality of life, and prioritized outcomes for early intervention in families of children with ASD [22]. Further comparisons are impossible because the scale was not yet used together with selected factors (e.g., parent gender) in other studies.

A strong negative correlation between AFEQ total score and WEMWBS score is evidence which shows better autism family experience correlation with higher well-being. This replicates the correlation found within the UK sample [22] and offers further evidence of the external validity of the relatively new AFEQ measure. Moreover, this finding showed that parents who have better mental well-being have better family experience of ASD and vice versa. Other studies have highlighted that stress harms caregiving experiences and feelings about being a parent [33, 34].

3.4.1 Limitations

One limitation of this study is that many participating parents were recruited through an NGO supporting autistic people and their parents. Therefore, these parents may receive more support regarding their child with ASD than is typical in Slovenia. The data may not represent the full range and diversity of difficulties related to ASD. The AFEQ is a relatively new tool, and there is a minimal number of cross-cultural studies to compare our results. However, it is currently being used in several cultural contexts, so understanding how the tool works across contexts will increase. Furthermore, the UK study sample [22] was larger ($n = 145$) than the sample in our study ($n = 101$). Future studies are needed to check the validity of the AFEQ scale among different environments and study samples.

3.5 Conclusion

The findings highlight the importance of family and parental well-being. Parenting can be stressful, especially for parents caring for a child with ASD. There were high levels of dissatisfaction with healthcare support within this Slovenian sample of parents of children with ASD. When parents have good support in the healthcare system, they maintain or improve their mental well-being. The findings highlight the importance of parental well-being by working outside the home and having time to yourself. Thus, it is very important that they have appropriate support from other family members and healthcare workers. Healthcare workers must be competent and have the knowledge, skills, and attitude for informing, teaching, and helping parents of children with ASD.

References

[1]   American Psychiatric Association. Diagnostic and statistical manual of mental disorders (DSM-V). 5th ed. Arlington, American Psychiatric Publishing, 2013.
[2]   Herrema R, Garland D, Osborne M, Freeston M, Honey E, Rodgers J. Mental wellbeing of family members of autistic adults. J Autism Dev Disord, 2017, 47(11), 3589–3599.
[3]   Miranda A, Mira A, Berenguer C, Rosello B, Baixauli I. Parenting stress in mothers of children with autism without intellectual disability. Mediation of behavioral problems and coping strategies. Front Psychol, 2019, 10, 464.
[4]   Catalano D, Holloway L, Mpofu E. Mental health interventions for parent carers of children with autistic spectrum disorder: Practice guidelines from a Critical Interpretive Synthesis (CIS) systematic review. Int J Environ Res Public Health, 2018, 15, 2.
[5]   Giallo R, Wood CE, Jellett R, Porter R. Fatigue, well-being and parental self-efficacy in mothers of children with an autism spectrum disorder. Autism, 2013, 17(4), 465–480.
[6]   DePape AM, Lindsay S. Parents' experiences of caring for a child with autism spectrum disorder. Qual Health Res, 2015, 25(4), 569–583.
[7]   Fairthorne J, de Klerk N, Leonard H. Brief report: Burden of care in mothers of children with autism spectrum disorder or intellectual disability. J Autism Dev Disord, 2016, 46(3), 1103–1109.
[8]   Keenan BM, Newman LK, Gray KM, Rinehart NJ. Parents of children with ASD experience more psychological distress, parenting stress, and attachment-related anxiety. J Autism Dev Disord, 2016, 46(9), 2979–2991.
[9]   Pisula E, Porębowicz-Dörsmann A. Family functioning, parenting stress and quality of life in mothers and fathers of Polish children with high functioning autism or Asperger syndrome. PLoS One, 2017, 12(10), e0186536.
[10] MacKean G. Mental health and well-being in postsecondary education settings: A literature and environmental scan to support planning and action in Canada. Canadian association of college and university student services, 2011. (Available from: http://www.cacuss.ca/_Library/documents/Post_Sec_Final_Report_June6.pdf).
[11] Isnis Isa M. Singapore mental well-being scales for children & youth, 2013. (Available from: https://www.imh.com.sg/uploadedFiles/Clinical_Services/Community-based_Services/REACH/Isnis-Singapore-Mental-Wellbeing-Scale.pdf).

[12] Ludlow A, Skelly C, Rohleder P. Challenges faced by parents of children diagnosed with autism spectrum disorder. J Health Psychol, 2012, 17(5), 702–711.

[13] Nomaguchi KM. Parenthood and psychological well-being: Clarifying the role of child age and parent-child relationship quality. Soc Sci Res, 2012, 41(2), 489–498.

[14] Da Paz NS, Siegel B, Coccia MA, Epel ES. Acceptance or despair? Maternal adjustment to having a child diagnosed with autism. J Autism Dev Disord, 2018, 48(6), 1971–1981.

[15] Vohra R, Madhavan S, Sambamoorthi U, St Peter C. Access to services, quality of care, and family impact for children with autism, other developmental disabilities, and other mental health conditions. Autism, 2014, 18(7), 815–826.

[16] Padden C, James JE. Stress among parents of children with and without autism spectrum disorder: A comparison involving physiological indicators and parent self-reports. J Dev Phys Disabil, 2017, 29(4), 567–586.

[17] Jamison JM, Fourie E, Siper PM, Trelles MP, George-Jones J, Buxbaum Grice A, et al. Examining the efficacy of a family peer advocate model for black and hispanic caregivers of children with autism spectrum disorder. J Autism Dev Disord, 2017, 47(5), 1314–1322.

[18] Cidav Z, Marcus SC, Mandell DS. Implications of childhood autism for parental employment and earnings. Pediatrics, 2012, 129(4), 617–623.

[19] Becerra TA, Massolo ML, Yau VM, Owen-Smith AA, Lynch FL, Crawford PM, et al. A survey of parents with children on the autism spectrum: Experience with services and treatments. Perm J, 2017, 21, 16–19.

[20] Schmidt J, Schmidt M, Brown I. Quality of life among families of children with intellectual disabilities: A Slovene study. J Policy Pract Intellect Disabil, 2017, 14(1), 87–102.

[21] Mertan E, Croucher L, Shafran R, Bennett SD. An investigation of the information provided to the parents of young people with mental health needs on an internet forum. Internet Interv, 2021, 23, 100353.

[22] Leadbitter K, Aldred C, McConachie H, Le Couteur A, Kapadia D, Charman T, et al. The Autism Family Experience Questionnaire (AFEQ): An ecologically-valid, parent-nominated measure of family experience, quality of life and prioritised outcomes for early intervention. J Autism Dev Disord, 2018, 48(4), 1052–1062.

[23] Beaton D, Bombardier C, Guillemin F, Ferraz MB. Recommendations for the cross-cultural adaptation of the DASH & QuickDASH outcome measures. IWH, 2007, 1(1), 1–45.

[24] Tennant R, Hiller L, Fishwick R, Platt S, Joseph S, Weich S, et al. The Warwick-Edinburgh Mental Well-being Scale (WEMWBS): Development and UK validation. Health Qual Life Outcomes, 2007, 5(1), 63.

[25] R Development Core Team. A language and environment for statistical computing. Vienna, R Foundation for Statistical Computing, 2005.

[26] National Health Service. Well-being self-assessment, 2011. (Available from: http://www.nhs. uk/Tools/Documents/Well-being%20self-assesment.htm).

[27] Evans JD. Straightforward statistics for the behavioral sciences. Thomson Brooks/Cole Publishing Co, 1996.

[28] Hitchcott PK, Fastame MC, Ferrai J, Penna MP. Psychological well-being in Italian families: An exploratory approach to the study of mental health across the adult life span in the blue zone. Eur J Psychol, 2017, 13(3), 441–454.

[29] Davis III TE, Hess JA, Moree BN, Fodstad JC, Dempsey T, Jenkins WS, et al. Anxiety symptoms across the lifespan in people diagnosed with autistic disorder. Res Autism Spectr Disord, 2011, 5(1), 112–118.

[30] Lai WW, Goh TJ, Oei TP, Sung M. Coping and well-being in parents of children with Autism Spectrum Disorders (ASD). J Autism Dev Disord, 2015, 45(8), 2582–2593.

[31] van Bourgondien ME, Dawkins T, Marcus L. Families of adults with autism spectrum disorders. In: Volkmar FR, Reichow B, McPartland JC, Eds. Adolescents and adults with autism spectrum disorders. New York, Springer, 2014, 15–40.
[32] Macdonald OF. Putting the puzzle together: Factors related to emotional well-being in parents of children with Autism Spectrum Disorders, 2011.
[33] Benson PR. Coping, distress, and well-being in mothers of children with autism. Res Autism Spectr Disord, 2010, 4(2), 217–228.
[34] Benson PR, Karlof KL. Anger, stress proliferation, and depressed mood among parents of children with ASD: A longitudinal replication. J Autism Dev Disord, 2009, 39(2), 350–362.

Dominika Vrbnjak, Dušica Pahor, Majda Pajnkihar

4 The relationship between perceptions of caring relationships, person-centred climate, and medication administration in nursing: a mixed-methods study

Abstract: Medication administration errors are a severe safety issue, especially in hospitals. Analysis of the medication errors process is needed for quality care and patient safety. Previous studies show positive outcomes related to caring culture in nursing, such as patient satisfaction. However, little is known about the relationships between caring culture and medication administration errors. Therefore, we aimed to analyze the causes of medication administration errors, reasons for not reporting them, the estimated percentage of reported medication administration errors, and how this correlates with perceptions of caring cultures among nursing staff in hospital settings. We have conducted a sequential explanatory mixed-methods study. Quantitative data gathering included five psychometrically sound questionnaires with 790 nurses and nursing assistants working in 69 surgical and internal wards in 11 Slovenian hospitals. Perceptions of medication administration errors were measured using the Medication Administration Error Survey. Caring relationships were measured using the Caring Factor Surveys. The person-centred climate was measured using a Person-centred climate questionnaire – staff version. We have used descriptive and inferential statistics to describe and interpret data. Grounded theory was used in the qualitative strand. Data collected with open-ended questions and semi-structured interviews were coded using OpenCode 3.6 software. Quantitative and qualitative findings were integrated at the interpretation level. Quantitative results showed that medication administration errors mainly occur due to nurses' resources and knowledge, working processes, and communication with physicians. Participants believed that underreporting is the result of fear and inadequate response. Perceptions of person-centred climate, safety climate, caring of provider, and caring by manager were linked with more significant medication error reporting. Core category lack of caring for patient safety with several categories emerged from qualitative analysis. The study showed a lack of caring relationships at the organizational and individual levels, various complex organizational and personal factors, errors occurrence, and underreporting. A caring culture was found to be the basis for safety; however, there are many other, mostly organizational, system issues. There is a need for a systematic approach in hospital settings.

Keywords: Medication administration errors, safety, reporting, caring culture, nursing

4.1 Introduction

The World Health Organization launched the global initiative *Medication Without Harm* to decrease severe preventable medication harm by half over five years [1]. Medication errors are preventable events related to causing unnecessary harm, costs, and even deaths [2]. The worldwide cost of medication errors has been estimated at 42 billion US dollars yearly [1]. For example, England counts 37 million medication errors each year, costing their health care system over 98 million GBP. Medication errors are causing or contributing to between 712 and 1,708 deaths. Prevalence and cost analysis of medication errors in Slovenia have not been done [3].

Reporting medication errors is essential for quality care and patient safety [4–6]. Nurses are accountable for reporting, and only by reporting the cause analyses is possible [5]. However, more medication administration errors occur than reported [4, 7], and underreporting results from various individual and system reasons [4, 8, 9]. Research shows reporting rates from 10 to 67% of actual cases [4, 9–11].

Safety culture is frequently addressed for improving patient safety [12, 13]. Some research shows positive relationships between safety culture and medication error reporting; however, other possible variables should be considered [12]. The caring concept is the foundation for quality of care [14–17] and has been theoretically linked to patient safety [14, 15, 18]. Errors are not always the result of a lack of knowledge and skills but also uncaring behaviour [19]. As nurses should perform person-centred care with a caring approach [20], person-centredness is closely linked to caring [20, 21]. Especially supportive environment such as a person-centred climate is needed to support the patient as a person. Individuals and their needs and beliefs should be the centre of attention and care [22, 23]. Both concepts are essential in nursing care; however, to our knowledge, no studies were conducted examining relationships between caring relationships, person-centred climate, and medication error administration.

4.1.1 Background

There are many causes of medication administration errors and these could be defined as individual or system factors [6]. Some of the critical causes highlighted by nursing staff are the lack of knowledge of nurses [6, 24], disruptions and interruptions in work [25], ineffective oral and written communication, and fatigue [26]. Errors also occur due to non-compliance with recommended guidelines or standards [25] and various drug delivery systems [27].

Open and honest disclosure is crucial to patient safety. Medication administration error reporting is mainly influenced by organizational barriers like culture, error reporting systems and management. However, personal and professional characteristics like fear, accountability, and nurses' attributes influence reporting [4]. Researching the reporting errors is vital for better patient safety. However, it is an under-researched topic in Slovenia [3, 28, 29]. Slovene hospital records show that only a few medication errors are reported yearly [28, 30], pointing to the possibility of a high underreporting rate.

In her Theory of Human Caring, Jean Watson describes nursing as person-centred transpersonal caring [31]. Caring relationships include relationships with the patient and outside nurse–patient relationships such as co-workers and managers [32]. When nurses have positive perceptions of caring in their work environment, this improves the perception of caring in patients [33]. To be a caring person, one should be cared for and have established caring relationships with all persons one works with [34, 35]. Nurse managers have an essential role in creating a caring environment and caring relationships with their staff [36–38]. Caring managers promote values of person-centred care, compassion, respect, and caring for the patient. They are aware that errors can happen to the best nurses, so they treat errors confidentially and constructively [34]. They are also strongly committed to creating a working environment that allows nurses to establish genuine, caring relationships with patients [37]. Nurses spend much of their time with their nurse peers; therefore, these relationships could also create a caring environment [39].

It has been established that caring is significantly linked to patient well-being and satisfaction [17, 40, 41] and nurse mental well-being [40], but there is limited research and evidence on its impact on patient safety. Glennon Kempf [42] researched caring leadership characteristics of nurse managers and patient satisfaction and quality of care and found no statistically significant relationships, possibly because of the small sample size and inclusion of only some nursing-sensitive indicators. Relationships between nurse-sensitive indicators and nurse caring behaviours were studied by Burt [43], who also found no significant relationship, possibly due to the small sample size and underreporting of adverse occurrences. However, both Glennon Kempf [42] and Burt [43] focused only on a selected type of caring relationship, either caring relationships with managers or relationship with the patients.

Person-centred care is also associated with quality of care [44–46] and focuses on an individual person's perspective [47]. Attributes of nurses and the care environment should be considered when delivering person-centred outcomes [48]. Edvardsson et al. [22] found that especially psychosocial dimensions of care environments support the provision of person-centred care. An important indicator of caring environments is the perception of a person-centred climate [49]. Researchers have established a link between person-centredness and quality of care, but limited research on how person-centred climate relates to organizational quality indicators [50].

Caring for patients, caring relationships with managers and coworkers, and a person-centred climate are essential elements of caring culture [30, 51]. Research on caring and person-centred climate could lead to greater safety and quality; however, limited research supports a positive relationship between caring relationships, person-centred climate, and medication error administration in nursing.

4.2 The study

4.2.1 Aim

We aimed to determine the causes and reporting of medication administration errors, reasons for not reporting them, the estimated percentage of reported medication administration errors and how this correlates with perceptions of caring culture.

4.2.2 Design

We have conducted a multi-centre descriptive study using a sequential explanatory mixed-methods design.

4.2.3 Setting and sample

The study population in the quantitative strand consisted of nurses and nursing assistants employed in internal and surgical units in hospital settings. Twelve Slovene hospitals have at least one or more medical and surgical units [50]. Of those 12, one hospital declined to participate, and 69 units in two university medical centres and seven general hospitals were included in the research. Convenience sampling was used and we conducted a priori sample size calculation with G-power (version 3.0.10) in a pilot study of 120 nursing employees of surgical and medical units in two hospitals. Assuming a power of 95% and 5% type I error rate, an adequate sample size calculation resulted in 115 nursing employees [30]. However, as hospitals were interested in the study, we decided to invite all nurses and nursing assistants responsible for enteral or parenteral medication administration who were working in a morning or afternoon shift and willing to participate in the study on a selected day when questionnaires were distributed. Nurse managers were excluded, as they rarely administer medications [29, 50]. Of the 1,295 distributed questionnaires, 790 were returned, giving a 61% response rate. Of 790 respondents, 382 answered at least one open question in the questionnaire (48.4% response).

In the qualitative strand, purposive sampling was used. Six head nurses of hospitals, clinics, departments, and wards who have knowledge and experience and come from different backgrounds and were able to help develop concepts and understand the research issues were included.

4.2.4 Data collection and analysis

Quantitative strand

We collected data from October 2015 to March 2016. Questionnaires were administered to nursing employees on a selected day by a researcher, nurse manager or hospital's nurse research coordinator, depending on hospital research policy. Nursing employees returned questionnaires in sealed envelopes or to a designated box.

Hospital, unit, and nursing employees' characteristics include hospital and unit size (number of beds and number of employees), age, sex, educational level, unit, number of years working as a nurse or nursing assistant, and number of years in the current unit was collected.

Medication administration error was measured using the Medication Administration Error Survey (MAE) Wakefield, Uden-Holman [52]. The MAE consists of three parts: reasons why medication errors occur (29 statements, 6-item Likert scale), why medication errors are not reported (16 statements, 6-item Likert scale), and estimated percentage of medication errors reported [11, 53–56]. Slovene versions of questionnaires were translated and evaluated for their psychometric properties in previous studies [29, 30, 50].

Three versions of the Caring Factor Survey (CFS) were used to measure caring relationships as perceived by nursing employees: 20-item Caring Factor Survey – Care Provider Version (CFS-CP) [57], 10-item CFS – Caring of Manager (CFS-CM) [58], and CFS – Caring for Co-workers (CFS-CC) [59]. All three instruments are designed as a 7-item Likert Scale.

Perception of how a climate of hospital environment from nursing employees is viewed as person-centred can be measured using a 14-item Person-centred climate questionnaire – staff version (PCQ-S), by Edvardsson et al. [22]. The questionnaire is designed as a 6-item Likert scale that can explore how employees experience the environment or climate of hospital settings as person-centred [23, 60, 61]. Using descriptive and inferential statistics, statistical analysis was done using IBM SPSS Statistics (Version 20.0. for Windows).

Qualitative strand

To facilitate the interpretation of the data, we also added open-ended questions related to researched constructs in the quantitative strand.

After quantitative analysis, sequenced data collection using semi-structured interviews was carried out in 2016. The interview guide was prepared based on quantitative data analysis [30]. The recorded interviews lasted up to 1 h and were later transcribed. We used field notes and theoretical and analytical memos to support the data analysis process. The qualitative data analysis was performed using Corbin and Strauss's coding paradigm [62]. It was supported using OpenCode 3.6 software [63].

Data integration

Integration of quantitative and qualitative data was carried out using the grounded theory approach by Corbin and Strauss (2015) and a discussion of the findings.

4.2.5 Ethical considerations

Republic of Slovenia National Medical Ethics Committee permitted to conduct the study (no. 127/07/14).

4.3 Results

4.3.1 Quantitative strand

The participants were 790 nursing staff with a mean age of 37.58 and mean years' experience of 16.19. Most were female (n = 684, 86.6%), nursing assistants 48.8% (n = 378), followed by nurses with diploma degree (n = 323; 40.9%); 64.2% (n = 507) were employed on surgical and 35.2% (n = 278) on internal wards.

Table 4.1 shows descriptive statistics for components of the MAE questionnaire, reasons for medication administration error occurrence and reasons for not being reported: 455 (70.8%) respondents perceived that all errors were reported at 0–60%, and 188 (29.2%) considered that all errors were reported at 61–100%.

For PCQ-S, the mean value was 4.39 (SD = 0.86). Mean values for subscales climate of safety, the climate of community and climate of everydayness were 4.68 (SD = 0.89), 4.36 (SD = 1.14), 3.67 (SD = 1.15), and 4.39 (SD = 0.86), respectively. The mean value for CFS-CP was 5.84 (SD = 0.76), for CFS-CM 5.84 (SD = 1.40), and for CFS-CC 5.04 (SD = 1.24).

Tab. 4.1: Reasons why medication errors occur and are not reported.

Reasons why medication administration errors occur	*n*	Mean	Standard deviation
Human resources and work processes	781	3.93	1.05
Physician communication	782	3.86	1.02
Knowledge	781	3.85	0.94
Medication packaging	782	3.81	1.30
Individual causes	783	2.62	0.85
Pharmacy processes	780	2.07	0.91
Reasons why medication administration errors are not reported			
Response	759	3.54	1.17
Fear	763	2.80	1.08
Reporting process	762	2.72	0.94

n, number of participants.

Table 4.2 shows relationships between perceptions of caring relationships with patients, co-workers and managers, person-centred climate, and medication administration error reporting.

Tab. 4.2: Perceptions of caring relationships with patients, co-workers and managers, person-centred climate, and medication administration error reporting.

Scale/subscale	% of reported MAE	Mean rank	*n*	Mann–Whitney *U*	*Z*	*p*	*n*
PCQ-S	0–60%	310.03	452	46,769.00	2.124	0.034*	639
	61–100%	344.10	187				
Climate of safety	0–60%	307.38	452	47,964.50	2.696	0.007*	639
	61–100%	350.49	187				
Climate of everydayness	0–60%	311.99	452	45,884.00	1.710	0.087	639
	61–100%	339.37	187				
Climate of community	0–60%	317.27	452	43,497.00	0.585	0.559	639
	61–100%	326.60	187				

Tab. 4.2 (continued)

Scale/subscale	% of reported MAE	Mean rank	n	Mann–Whitney U	Z	p	n
CFS-CP	0–60%	305.15	447	46,869.50	2.530	0.011*	633
	61–100%	345.49	186				
CFS-CM	0–60%	307.31	448	46,678.50	2.277	0.023*	635
	61–100%	343.62	187				
CFS-CC	0–60%	312.05	449	43,977.50	1.169	0.243	634
	61–100%	330.72	185				

*Statistical significance at ≤ 0.05; %, percent; CFS-CC, Caring Factor Survey-Caring for Co-workers; CFS-CM, Caring Factor Survey-Caring of Manager; CFS-CP, Caring Factor Survey-Care Provider version; n, number of participants; p, statistical significance; PCQ-S, person-centred climate questionnaire – staff version; Z, Z-score.

4.3.2 Qualitative strand

Six categories were constructed by researchers in the process of analysis of open-ended questions: perceptions of medication administration errors; organizational and individual factors of medication administration errors; inconsistent perception of reporting medication administration errors; organizational and individual factors for not reporting medication administration errors; improving medication safety and caring for patient and caring culture.

The main category "lack of caring for safety" was constructed. Due to a lack of caring at the organizational and individual level, the respondents described the practice as one where medication errors occur and are underreported. Respondents believe that we do not know how many errors happen in practice. They also provided different definitions of what constitutes medication administration error. Errors are the result of various complex organizational (staff workload, medication administration process, management support, and interprofessional collaboration) and individual factors (knowledge and training, caring). These are also not fully reported due to various organizational (culture, system, and management of reporting medication administration errors) and individual factors (fear, responsibility, and caring).

The respondents pointed out the shortcomings in the existing work organization, the workload, and the lack of staff. For example: "Mistakes happen because employees are mostly very busy. . . ."

Due to the workload and lack of staff, there are shortcomings in the medication administration process; there is a pre-preparation of medicines, disregard of competencies, and the use of the so-called "notebook therapy" for orientation on how much and which medications are needed on nursing trolleys. Disruptions at work also contribute to errors. Some medications cannot be delivered on time and are prepared in advance, mainly for the morning shift. It is a practice that everyone is aware of but reluctant to discuss. For the same reasons, nursing assistants often administer intravenous therapy. For instance: "Therapy is not prepared in advance . . . except on weekends and at night . . . but not officially. . ." and "Too many times something interrupts you at work . . . in the meantime, someone comes and orders you something, one physician this, another nurse this, the phone, a third . . . ."

Another important factor the respondents pointed out was the lack of interprofessional cooperation with pharmacists and physicians, especially concerning generic medications. There are lists of interchangeable medications in the wards, but they are not the best solution. One respondent recounted their experience this way: " in the morning when I order medication, I don't know which parallel I'm getting. And when that parallel comes, the physician should, according to all the rules, write it on the patient therapy sheet . . . but he won't come out of the operating room because of that. . .".

Respondents highlighted the lack of knowledge about medications and patient safety during education and the lack of training for employees. New employees are a problem because they lack knowledge and experience, and it is necessary to emphasize the need for continuous improvement and training. One expressed problem: "I did not acquire this necessary knowledge during the education, I acquired the knowledge later in practice . . . but the management and supervisors must pay enough attention to this and take care of continuous education, improvement and then transfer what has been learned into practice. . . ."

The respondents highlighted caring as an important factor, namely caring for safety, quality, professional work, and compliance with standards. Failure to do so may result in errors. For instance: "We can't work safely without caring for patient . . . if you don't have morale, ethics in you. . . ." Respondents believe that caring has a psychological and technical dimension, and they see it as holistic and individual care that requires a mutual partnership. Some expressed beliefs: "Caring means to me that you take care of the patient from all perspectives, to embrace him as a whole. . ." and "To act the way you would like to be cared. . .". They believe that caring is something you are born with but can be learned as well. It is a personal quality that an individual acquires in a family environment and later builds in the context of education and the workplace: "Caring for another person is a reflection of one's upbringing and the environment (family) from which one comes, and then you constantly build on it during education, employment, and function . . . ." Caring for an individual is not enough to ensure safety; one must perceive caring in co-workers, superiors, and the entire work environment. For instance: "it's not just caring for the patient, there's also caring for the co-worker, caring in the work environment, I often miss that. . .". Even though according to the respondents, caring is the foundation and precondition for safety, they point out that other factors also lead to errors.

Organizational and individual factors for underreporting of medication administration errors

Respondents highlighted a silent culture, where medication errors are not discussed. For instance: "What is not reported does not exist. . . ." Reporting also differs slightly from one institution to another. In general, they believe that we are looking for individual culprits in our environments and punishing them. System approach and punitive culture pervade. One respondent expressed concern: "They are still trying to find out who is guilty, point the finger at one person and punish them . . . if an error happens, someone is punished. . . ." The reporting system is anonymous; errors are reported to superiors, and a root cause analysis and corrective action are implemented. However, despite the anonymous system, the identity of the culprit can be revealed. There is also a problem with the complexity of the reporting system and the burden to the employee.

Respondents predict fear as the main reason why errors are not reported. Fear stems primarily from a punitive culture. Employees are afraid of the consequences and the punishment that may follow. They are also ashamed of errors and worried about their careers and their co-workers' thinking about them. They also fear the response from patients and their families. Error reporting can also be negatively affected by media reactions. For example: "That fear, what will happen, what others will think of me, what if the patient finds out, what if it is written down somewhere, how it will affect my career . . . and there is also media. . . ." Underreporting can also be due to a lack of responsibility of the individual; also, one must acknowledge and be aware of the error.

4.4 Discussion

Medication administration errors are a safety issue, and organizational and individual factors influence their occurrence. Organizational factors include personal factors, work processes, medication delivery processes, communication with physicians, medicines, pharmacists, management support, knowledge and skills. Individual factors include personal characteristics and individual and patient factors. Nursing employees perceive errors as something negative, and the inconsistency of definitions is worrying, as it can affect reporting. Underreporting is also influenced by several organizational and individual causes, including response, communication processes and culture, fear, responsibility, and professional and personal characteristics. Elements of caring culture are associated with medication error reporting. Caring culture is the foundation for patient safety; however, other factors influence medication administration errors and reporting.

Our findings align with previous work examining the causes [64] and reporting of medication administration errors [65]. We found very problematic generic substitutions. Respondents are concerned about the situation; they report a lack of knowledge and skills. Nurse managers should implement strategies to address this potential risk of error. Some suggest that standardized labelling and information about medication may reduce nurse time in the medication administration process [66]. Essential is adequate support from pharmacists and efficient communication with physicians [26]. Lack of staff and high workload are common factors for errors in existing literature [67]. Managers and policymakers should evaluate and implement strategies to overcome staff shortages and manage increased workloads effectively without increasing staff.

Caring was perceived as an holistic and individual approach that requires mutual interpersonal relationships, which is also in line with other findings [68]. Nursing includes technical and expressive skills and knowledge [69]. Respondents perceived caring as providing for physical needs and respecting the person as a whole, thus providing for spiritual needs and creating positive energy. Caring is about ensuring dignity, inspiring hope, empathy and compassion and caring for others as you want others to take care of you. Caring is perceived as a moral and ethical act or as Watson claims – a moral imperative [70].

Respondents also believe that caring is the foundation for safety and quality; however, caring behaviours of all nurses and managers and a caring environment are needed. It is difficult to discuss findings because relationships between caring [30], person-centredness [71] and medication administration are under-researched. However, it is well established that organizational culture and safety climate impact medication administration error occurrence and reporting. Leadership management and interprofessional relationships with colleagues are also critical [72, 73].

Readers should interpret findings with caution due to convenience sampling, self-reported data collection techniques, and cross-sectional design. Social-desirability bias is possible. The study should be replicated, mainly as we have conducted a study prior Covid-19 pandemic, which has caused nursing additional staffing shortages and other challenges [74]. Further studies should evaluate cause-effect relationships using more robust research designs. Interventions for improving safety need to be implemented and evaluated. There is a possibility of exploring relationships between caring culture and other nurse-sensitive indicators, like patient falls and bed sores. Nurse education and training interventions can actively improve patient safety. Stronger emphasis on acquiring knowledge of pharmacology, mathematical skills in calculating drug doses, critical thinking and clinical decision-making, clinical judgment, effective teamwork and communication, and the prevention and reporting of errors are needed.

4.5 Conclusion

Our study highlights the lack of caring in medication administration, especially at the system level. Several complex organizational and personal factors influence medication administration errors. Medication error reporting is influenced by caring culture. Hospital settings require a systematic approach to reduce medication administration errors. Nurses will report errors in culture, where caring is nurtured and when not perceiving fear and blame.

References

[1] World Health Organization. Medication without harm – global patient safety challenge on medication safety. Geneva, World Health Organization, 2017.

[2] Ciapponi A, Fernandez Nievas SE, Seijo M, Rodríguez MB, Vietto V, García-Perdomo HA, et al. Reducing medication errors for adults in hospital settings. Cochrane Database Syst Rev, 2021, 11(11), Cd009985.

[3] Robida A. Kriminalizacija človeških napak v zdravstvu: Rešitev ali poguba za paciente? Isis, 2012, 17–23.

[4] Vrbnjak D, Denieffe S, O'Gorman C, Pajnkihar M. Barriers to reporting medication errors and near misses among nurses: A systematic review. Int J Nurs Stud, 2016, 63, 162–178.

[5] Haw C, Stubbs J, Dickens GL. Barriers to the reporting of medication administration errors and near misses: An interview study of nurses at a psychiatric hospital. J Psychiatr Ment Health Nurs, 2014.

[6] Brady A, Malone A, Fleming S. A literature review of the individual and systems factors that contribute to medication errors in nursing practice. J Nurs Manag, 2009, 17(6), 679–697.

[7] Hajibabaee F, Joolaee S, Peyravi H, Alijany-Renany H, Bahrani N, Haghani H. Medication error reporting in Tehran: A survey. J Nurs Manag, 2014, 22(3), 304–310.

[8] Parry AM, Barriball KL, While AE. Factors contributing to Registered Nurse medication administration error: A narrative review. Int J Nurs Stud, 2015, 52(1), 403–420.

[9] Keers RN, Williams SD, Cooke J, Ashcroft DM. Prevalence and nature of medication administration errors in health care settings: A systematic review of direct observational evidence. Ann Pharmacother, 2013, 47(2), 237–256.

[10] Berdot S, Gillaizeau F, Caruba T, Prognon P, Durieux P, Sabatier B. Drug administration errors in hospital inpatients: A systematic review. PLoS One, 2013, 8(6), e68856.

[11] Wakefield DS, Wakefield BJ, Borders T, Uden-Holman T, Blegen M, Vaughn T. Understanding and comparing differences in reported medication administration error rates. Am J Med Qual, 1999, 14(2), 73–80.

[12] Groves PS. The relationship between safety culture and patient outcomes: Results from pilot meta-analyses. West J Nurs Res, 2014, 36(1), 66–83.

[13] Kagan I, Barnoy S. Organizational safety culture and medical error reporting by Israeli nurses. J Nurs Scholarsh, 2013, 45(3), 273–280.

[14] Duffy JR, Hoskins LM. The quality-caring model: Blending dual paradigms. ANS Adv Nurs Sci, 2003, 26(1), 77–88.

[15] Watson J. Caring science and human caring theory: Transforming personal and professional practices of nursing and health care. J Health Hum Serv Adm, 2009, 31(4), 466–482.

[16] McCance TV. Caring in nursing practice: The development of a conceptual framework. Res Theory Nurs Pract, 2003, 17(2), 101–116.

[17] Pajnkihar M, Stiglic G, Vrbnjak D. The concept of Watson's carative factors in nursing and their (dis)harmony with patient satisfaction. PeerJ, 2017, 5, e2940.

[18] Watson J. Nursing: Human science and human care: A theory of nursing. Boston, Jones & Bartlett Learning, 1999.

[19] Tzeng HM. Nurses' caring attitude: Fall prevention program implementation as an example of its importance. Nurs Forum, 2011, 46(3), 137–145.

[20] McCance T, Slater P, McCormack B. Using the caring dimensions inventory as an indicator of person-centred nursing. J Clin Nurs, 2009, 18(3), 409–417.

[21] Hesselink G, Kuis E, Pijnenburg M, Wollersheim H. Measuring a caring culture in hospitals: A systematic review of instruments. BMJ Open, 2013, 3(9), e003416.

[22] Edvardsson D, Sandman PO, Rasmussen B. Swedish language person-centred climate questionnaire – patient version: Construction and psychometric evaluation. J Adv Nurs, 2008, 63(3), 302–309.

[23] Edvardsson D, Sandman PO, Rasmussen B. Construction and psychometric evaluation of the Swedish language Person-centred Climate Questionnaire – staff version. J Nurs Manag, 2009, 17(7), 790–795.

[24] Cheragi MA, Manoocheri H, Mohammadnejad E, Ehsani SR. Types and causes of medication errors from nurse's viewpoint. Iran J Nurs Midwifery Res, 2013, 18(3), 228–231.

[25] Wondmieneh A, Alemu W, Tadele N, Demis A. Medication administration errors and contributing factors among nurses: A cross sectional study in tertiary hospitals, Addis Ababa, Ethiopia. BMC Nurs, 2020, 19(1), 4.

[26] Keers RN, Williams SD, Cooke J, Ashcroft DM. Causes of medication administration errors in hospitals: A systematic review of quantitative and qualitative evidence. Drug Saf, 2013, 36(11), 1045–1067.

[27] Kuitunen S, Niittynen I, Airaksinen M, Holmström AR. Systemic causes of in-hospital intravenous medication errors: A systematic review. J Patient Saf, 2021, 17(8), e1660–e8.

[28] Bračič A. Varnost na področju predpisovanja in ravnanja z zdravili kot kompleksen sistemski problem. Obzornik Zdravstvene Nege, 2011, 45(3), 213–218.

[29] Vrbnjak D, Pahor D, Štiglic G, Pajnkihar M. Content validity and internal reliability of Slovene version of medication administration error survey. Obzornik Zdravstvene Nege, 2016, 50(1), 20–40.

[30] Vrbnjak D. Caring for patient and safety in medication administration in nursing. Maribor, University of Maribor, 2017.

[31] Pajnkihar M, McKenna HP, Stiglic G, Vrbnjak D. Fit for practice: Analysis and evaluation of Watson's theory of human caring. Nurs Sci Q, 2017, 30(3), 243–252.

[32]   Nelson J, Watson J. Measuring caring: International research on caritas as healing. New York, Springer Publishing Company, 2012.

[33]   Berry DM, Kaylor MB, Church J, Campbell K, McMillin T, Wamsley R. Caritas and job environment: A replication of Persky et al. Contemp Nurse, 2013, 43(2), 237–243.

[34]   Brandt MA. Caring leadership: Secret and path to success. Nurs Manage, 1994, 25(8), 68–72.

[35]   Minnaar A. The views of nurses regarding caring in the workplace. Curationis, 2003, 26(1), 37–42.

[36]   Longo J. Acts of caring: Nurses caring for nurses. Holist Nurs Pract, 2011, 25(1), 8–16.

[37]   Dyess SM, Boykin A, Bulfin MJ. Hearing the voice of nurses in caring theory-based practice. Nurs Sci Q, 2013, 26(2), 167–173.

[38]   Carter LC, Nelson JL, Sievers BA, Dukek SL, Pipe TB, Holland DE. Exploring a culture of caring. Nurs Adm Q, 2008, 32(1), 57–63.

[39]   Kay Hogan B. Caring as a scripted discourse versus caring as an expression of an authentic relationship between self and other. Issues Ment Health Nurs, 2013, 34(5), 375–379.

[40]   Finfgeld-Connett D. Meta-synthesis of caring in nursing. J Clin Nurs, 2008, 17(2), 196–204.

[41]   Kaur D, Sambasivan M, Kumar N. Effect of spiritual intelligence, emotional intelligence, psychological ownership and burnout on caring behaviour of nurses: A cross-sectional study. J Clin Nurs, 2013, 22(21–22), 3192–3202.

[42]   Glennon Kempf S. Caring leadership attributes of RN CEOs and the relationship to patient satisfaction and quality [Ph.D.]. Ann Arbor, Capella University, 2011.

[43]   Burt KM. The relationship between nurse caring and selected outcomes of care in hospitalized older adults: Catholic University of America, 2007.

[44]   Edvardsson D, Winblad B, Sandman PO. Person-centred care of people with severe Alzheimer's disease: Current status and ways forward. Lancet Neurol, 2008, 7(4), 362–367.

[45]   Morgan S, Yoder LH. A concept analysis of person-centered care. J Holist Nurs, 2012, 30(1), 6–15.

[46]   Slater P, McCance T, McCormack B. The development and testing of the Person-centred Practice Inventory – Staff (PCPI-S). Int J Qual Health Care, 2017, 29(4), 541–547.

[47]   Slater P, McCance T, McCormack B. The development and testing of the Person-centred Practice Inventory – Staff (PCPI-S). Int J Qual Health Care, 2017, 29(4), 541–547.

[48]   McCance T, McCormack B, Slater P, McConnell D. Examining the theoretical relationship between constructs in the person-centred practice framework: A structural equation model. Int J Environ Res Public Health, 2021, 18(24), 13138.

[49]   Edvardsson JD, Sandman PO, Rasmussen BH. Sensing an atmosphere of ease: A tentative theory of supportive care settings. Scand J Caring Sci, 2005, 19(4), 344–353.

[50]   Vrbnjak D, Pahor D, Povalej Bržan P, Edvardsson D, Pajnkihar M. Psychometric testing of the Slovenian person-centred climate questionnaire – Staff version. J Nurs Manag, 2017, 25, 421–429.

[51]   Manley K. Insight into developing caring cultures: A review of the experience of the Foundation of Nursing Studies (FoNS). FoNS Centre for Nursing Innovation, 2013.

[52]   Wakefield BJ, Uden-Holman T, Wakefield DS. Development and validation of the medication administration error reporting survey. In: Advances in patient safety: From research to implementation (volume 4: programs, tools, and products) [Internet]. Rockville MD, Agency for Healthcare Research and Quality (US), 2005. Available from: http://www.ncbi.nlm.nih.gov/books/NBK20599/.

[53]   Wakefield BJ, Uden-Holman T, Wakefield DS. Development and Validation of the Medication Administration Error Reporting Survey. Advances in Patient Safety: From Research to Implementation (Volume 4: Programs, Tools, and Products). Henriksen K, Battles JB, Marks ES, Lewin DI, editors. Rockville MD2005 Feb.

[54] Wakefield BJ, Wakefield DS, Uden-Holman T, Blegen MA. Nurses' perceptions of why medication administration errors occur. Medsurg Nurs, 1998, 7(1), 39–44.

[55] Wakefield DS, Wakefield BJ, Uden-Holman T, Blegen MA. Perceived barriers in reporting medication administration errors. Best Pract Benchmarking Healthc, 1996, 1(4), 191–197.

[56] Wakefield DS, Wakefield BJ, Uden-Holman T, Borders T, Blegen M, Vaughn T. Understanding why medication administration errors may not be reported. Am J Med Qual, 1999, 14(2), 81–88.

[57] Johnson J. Creation of the Caring Factor Survey-Care Provider Version (CFS-CPV). In: Nelson J, Watson J, Eds. Masuring caring, International research on caritas as healing. New York, Springer Publishing Company, LLC, 2012, 40–46.

[58] Olender L, Phifer S. Development of the Caring Factor Survey-Caring of Manager (CFS-CM). In: Nelson J, Watson J, Eds. Masuring caring, International research on caritas as healing. New York, Springer Publishing Company, 2012, 57–63.

[59] Lawerence I, Kear M. The practice of loving kindness to self and others as perceived by nurses and patients in the cardiac interventional unit (CIU). In: Nelson J, Watson J, Eds. Masuring caring, International research on caritas as healing. New York, Springer Publishing Company, LLC, 2012.

[60] Bergland A, Kirkevold M, Edvardsson D. Psychometric properties of the Norwegian person-centred climate questionnaire from a nursing home context. Scand J Caring Sci, 2012, 26(4), 820–828.

[61] Edvardsson D, Koch S, Nay R. Psychometric evaluation of the English language Person-centred Climate Questionnaire–staff version. J Nurs Manag, 2010, 18(1), 54–60.

[62] Corbin J, Strauss A. Basics of qualitative research, tehniques and procedures for developing grounded theory. 4th ed. Thousand Oaks, California, SAGE Publications, Inc, 2015.

[63] ICT Services and System Development and Division of Epidemiology and Global Health. OpenCode 3.4. Umeå: Umeå University, 2013.

[64] Schroers G, Ross JG, Moriarty H. Nurses' perceived causes of medication administration errors: A qualitative systematic review. Jt Comm J Qual Patient Saf, 2020.

[65] Aljabari S, Kadhim Z. Common barriers to reporting medical errors. ScientificWorldJournal, 2021, 2021, 6494889.

[66] Garcia BH, Elenjord R, Bjornstad C, Halvorsen KH, Hortemo S, Madsen S. Safety and efficiency of a new generic package labelling: A before and after study in a simulated setting. BMJ Qual Saf, 2017, 26(10), 817–823.

[67] Jessurun JG, Hunfeld NGM, de Roo M, van Onzenoort HAW, van Rosmalen J, van Dijk M, et al. Prevalence and determinants of medication administration errors in clinical wards: A two-centre prospective observational study. J Clin Nurs, 2022.

[68] Wei H, Watson J. Healthcare interprofessional team members' perspectives on human caring: A directed content analysis study. Int J Nurs Sci, 2018, 6(1), 17–23.

[69] Li Y-S, Yu W-P, Yang B-H, Liu C-F. A comparison of the caring behaviours of nursing students and registered nurses: Implications for nursing education. J Clin Nurs, 2016, 25(21–22), 3317–3325.

[70] Watson J. Human caring science a theory of nursing. 2nd ed. Sudbury, Jones & Bartlett Learning, 2012.

[71] Rossiter C, Levett-Jones T, Pich J. The impact of person-centred care on patient safety: An umbrella review of systematic reviews. Int J Nurs Stud, 2020, 109, 103658.

[72] Jafree SR, Zakar R, Zakar MZ, Fischer F. Nurse perceptions of organizational culture and its association with the culture of error reporting: A case of public sector hospitals in Pakistan. BMC Health Serv Res, 2016, 16, 3.

[73] Alanazi FK, Sim J, Lapkin S. Systematic review: Nurses' safety attitudes and their impact on patient outcomes in acute-care hospitals. Nurs Open, 2022, 9(1), 30–43.

[74] Danesh MK, Garosi E, Golmohamadpour H. The COVID-19 Pandemic and nursing challenges: A review of the early literature. Work (Reading, Mass), 2021, 69(1), 23–36.

Mojca Dobnik, Mateja Lorber, Jackie Rowles

5 Pain monitoring analysis as a quality indicator: a retrospective study

Abstract

Introduction: To improve patient care and safety in hospital clinical settings, evidence-based and internationally comparable quality indicators (QI) need to be developed. The QI best demonstrates the pain management quality. This chapter aims to deliver an overview of the introduction of a pain monitoring QI and its use in clinical practice to evaluate the long-term monitoring effects of the pain QI in a clinical environment at one of the tertiary institutions in Slovenia.

Methods: A non-experimental quantitative study was carried out with a probabilistic random sample. Twenty per cent occupancy of the unit/department was analysed, and patient's documentation on the selected day at the tertiary institution for four consecutive years (2016 to 2019) was reviewed. Data were processed using bivariate and multivariate analysis.

Results: The study found a nonlinear pain monitoring increase across the five studied variables. The comparison between clinics did not show statistically significant differences ($F = 6.6$, $p = 0.14$) in the QI variables (pain assessment on admission, before and after therapy, appropriate analgesic, and daily assessment in patients with no pain).

Discussion and conclusion: The research provided insight into pain monitoring at a tertiary institution over 4 years. The data obtained might serve as the basis for surveys and policy-making at a national level, including protocol creation.

Keywords: Patient, pain, hospital

5.1 Introduction

Quality indicators (QI) were developed and are now being evolved by the Agency for Healthcare Research and Quality's (AHRQ). QI respond to the need for multidimensional, accessible criteria to improve performance in healthcare. The QI is a measurement tool to monitor, evaluate, and improve the quality of healthcare based on evidence-based practice [1]. In 1998, the American Nurses Association (ANA) designed the National Database of Nursing Quality Indicators (NDNQI). The database was created to meet the need to assess the impact of nursing on healthcare, the relationship between workload, workflow, and the relationship between nurses and patients. The connection between the nurse's recruitment and the outcomes and results in the work with patients was confirmed later. For the QI to be useful for monitoring the quality of care, it should be clinically relevant and reliable as well as valid [2].

Designing a QI is a multistep process that involves evaluating evidence if a particular indicator is used in clinical practice followed by pilot-testing of indicators. The National Database of Nursing Quality Indicators (NDNQI) continuously monitors and delivers validity and reliability tests. In nursing, a quality/outcome indicator is considered significant, if there is a connection or a multivariate link between single nursing aspects/process and the outcome. To evaluate a strong correlation between HR nursing structure and work outcomes, the NDNQI uses state-of-the-art methods, for example, mixed (hierarchical) model [3]. Evidence-based nursing used to be increasingly very important for patient outcomes. The status of patient care is now evaluated by QI [4].

Measuring outcome performance is crucial to improve quality as it provides information on current and previous performance to support further efforts for improvement. Therefore, the development and application of valid and reliable performance measurements are essential to improve the quality of care. This is one of the first steps in the improvement involving the selection, definition, and the use of performance indicators [5].

Patient safety indicators (PSIs) in AHRQ strengthen the clinical quality of the healthcare system. PSIs are a set of measures to coordinate quality improvement objectives throughout the system. They can be used to monitor trend data and provide root causes of any quality-related problem, even if documentation is the underlying problem. Without carefully prepared documentation, it is hard to identify true opportunities for quality improvement [6].

Many international organizations focus on pain management aiming to understand patients who are suffering from acute or chronic pain. Nursing personnel spend most of their time as the primary caregiver for the patient and are therefore crucial in the assessment and management of pain. In a hospital clinical setting, evidence-based and internationally comparable QI need to be developed to optimize patient care and safety. A reliable and valid QI for pain monitoring is the most suitable way to prove the quality of pain management. Pain assessment is crucial for effective pain management. Nurses have a unique role in the assessment of pain as they spend most of their time with the patient [7].

Pain that alleviates relatively quickly is referred to as acute pain. Prolonged pain is referred to as chronic or persistent pain. There are various definitions of acute and chronic pain. Some experts claim that acute pain lasts no longer than 30 days, while others argue that acute pain can be associated with any pain that resolves within 3 or 6 months. With its protective and healing function, acute pain serves as a useful survival mechanism. Chronic pain is most commonly described as pain lasting longer than 3–6 months or pain lasting longer than the normal healing time for the associate pathological process. Complex psychological and social factors may be encompassed in the pain [8]. Pain management in Europe focuses on the application of a biopsychosocial approach. This approach monitors the development of pain through a complex interaction of biological (genetics, biochemistry, etc.), psychological (mood, thoughts, beliefs), and social (cultural, family, socioeconomic, etc.) aspects. In this way, pain management consists of pharmacological (drugs), non-pharmacological therapies (exercise, cognitive behavioral therapy), patient education, invasive approaches, if necessary, and long-term pain management programs for people with chronic pain [8].

Patients referred to a facility with acute or chronic pain do not have any guarantee that their pain will be treated appropriately from an organizational perspective. In one study [9], 89% of hospitals declared to provide adequate pain management; however, only a few hospitals adhered to expert protocols. Considering the lack of adequate pain management, there are many concerns regarding the quality of monitoring. Thirty-eight per cent of patients report that their pain is not adequately managed [10]. Pain is the most common symptom in emergency care patients with more than half of patients reporting moderate pain intensity. Critically ill and intubated patients who are unable to communicate are even at greater risk of inadequate pain management [11]. Nurses lack knowledge about pain management, the complex practices in emergencies, factors affecting the detection, and nurses' judgment, assessment, and management of pain in critically ill patients are not well understood [12].

Casarett et al. [13] suggest that satisfaction with pain management can be measured and investigated reliably. Joy et al. [14] found that a multimodal training model improved the level of pain knowledge in nurses reporting patients pain. Patients expect rapid pain relief; however, this is not often achievable. Despite multiple inspiring developments in analgesic therapy, many obstacles remain in the assessment, monitoring, record keeping, and reassessment of pain [15].

5.1.1 Purpose and goals

The purpose of this study was to analyse pain monitoring data after QI introduction, following education of nursing staff, to identify the effectiveness of monitoring pain assessment in patients. The objective of the chapter is to evaluate the long-term monitoring of effects resulting from the introduction of the pain QI in a clinical setting in one of the tertiary facilities in Slovenia. A research question and hypothesis were developed as follows:

– Research question: Has the pain monitoring performance improved after the QI was introduced among nursing staff during the study period?
– Hypothesis: There are statistically significant differences in pain monitoring between departments within the institution.

5.2 Methods

A non-experimental quantitative research design – a retrospective study research design was applied.

5.2.1 Instrument description

Instead of collecting new data, information already obtained for monitoring the QI in the institution was used. The data was obtained using the following form: Control of compliance with the QI of pain monitoring in UKC Maribor. The form includes data on the organizational unit and the number of patients hospitalized on the selected day as well as the number of patient documentation included in the monitoring. In addition, the form includes the patient's ID number and six binary (Yes/No) items for pain monitoring: was the patient's pain assessed at admission; was the pain in patients, who did not report pain, assessed and recorded once a day; was pain assessment performed and documented before analgesia and one hour after analgesia, and was the patient-administered an appropriate analgesic according to the pain assessment. Initially, pilot monitoring was carried out in the first quarter of 2016. Monitoring documentation/review was repeated in autumn 2016 and 2017, 2018, and 2019.

5.2.2 Sample description

Monitoring was carried out on an ad-hoc documentation sample to conduct the analysis. Insight into the QI implementation, pain monitoring, and patient's health records (20% random sample all patients included for each unit) in the period from 2016 to 2019 enabled data collection. In 2016, the monitoring was carried out at 27 departments/units, and records of 142 patients were reviewed. In 2017, records of 181 patients in 31 departments/units were reviewed. In 2018, records of 158 patients at 31 departments/units were reviewed. In 2019, records of 102 patients at 21 departments/units were reviewed. Monitoring was carried out at the Division of Surgery, the Division of Internal Medicine, the Division of Gynecology and Obstetrics, and independent medical departments.

5.2.3 Research process and data processing description

We requested authorization to perform data analysis for the period from 2016 to 2019. SPPS version 20.0 (SPSS Inc., Chicago, IL, USA) was used for data analysis. Basic statistical calculations were used for individual variables as follows: arithmetic means/average, standard deviation, minimum, and maximum value, and percentages. ANOVA was used to determine statistically significant differences between divisions/independent medical departments/units. A statistical value less than 0.05 was considered significant.

5.3 Results

We found an increase in pain monitoring for all five items, except VAS monitoring at admission (90%) and one hour after the therapy was administered (71%) in 2018. Table 5.1 shows the pain monitoring analysis for the facility.

The analysis of results using ANOVA analysis for comparison between divisions showed no statistically significant differences ($F = 6.6$, $p = 0.14$) (Tab. 5.2).

Figure 5.1 shows the distribution of the variables between divisions across all five variables in the period from 2016 to 2019. This chart demonstrates the percentage of pain assessment at admission in the monitored period has been improving nonlinearly at the Division of Surgery (KK), increasing unevenly at Independent Medical Departments (SAM), and nonlinearly at the Division of Gynecology and Obstetrics (GIN), while this trend was not seen at the Division of Internal Medicine (KIM).

According to the tertiary level institution standard, it is necessary to check the presence of pain once a day in patients who do not report pain. During the follow-up period, monitoring improved nonlinearly at the Division of Surgery, nonlinearly at Independent Medical Departments, and nonlinearly at the Division of Gynecology and Obstetrics (GIN). A positive trend was also seen in the Division of Internal Medicine (KIM); however, this trend has not been maintained.

Pain assessment monitoring before analgesic administration improved nonlinearly across all divisions and independent medical departments. The monitored variable of appropriate analgesic administration improved nonlinearly across all divisions and independent medical departments. When monitoring the variable "assessment of pain after therapy administration" one can see the nonlinear improvement across all divisions and independent medical departments.

The Division of Surgery and Independent Medical Departments achieved improvement across all variables. The Division of Gynecology and Obstetrics achieved similar results; however, slightly lower percentage levels. At the Division of Internal Medicine, improvement was achieved in three of the five variables.

Tab. 5.1: Pain monitoring in the period from 2016 to 2019 at the facility.

Year	n	a	SD	Min/max	b	SD	Min/max	c	SD	Min/max	d	SD	Min/max	e	SD	Min/max
2016	142	78%	0.29	0/100	70%	0.29	0/100	57%	0.31	0/100	74%	0.24	0/100	39%	0.27	0/100
2017	181	91%	0.12	66/100	91%	0.14	50/100	87%	0.17	0/100	87%	0.18	0/100	82%	0.18	0/100
2018	158	90%	0.14	50/100	93%	0.12	50/100	83%	0.21	20/100	80%	0.34	20/100	71%	0.35	20/100
2019	102	96%	0.19	33/100	93%	0.26	57/100	100%	0.14	50/100	100%	0.5	10/100	100%	0.5	0/100

a, VAS at admission; b, once daily; c, before analgesics; d, appropriate analgesic administration; e, 1 h after analgesic administration; min/max, minimal value/maximal value; n, no. of records to be followed; SD, standard deviation.

Tab. 5.2: Results of a one-way analysis of variance (ANOVA).

Source of variation	Sum of square	Df	Mean square	F	p-Value
Between groups	8.208454603	15	0.547230307	6.594397517	0.14
Within groups	36.51301494	440	0.082984125		
Total	44.72146954	455			

df, degree of freedom; F, F-value; p, statistical significance.

5.4 Discussion

The research showed that in all five variables an average increase in pain assessment monitoring was noted in the tertiary institution, after QI and the training of head nurses were introduced, at the facility level. The research question "Has the pain monitoring performance improved after the quality indicator was introduced among nursing staff during the study period?" can be answered affirmatively. A prior study reported that nursing staff noticed improved pain monitoring over four weeks by 30% [16]. The literature review confirmed the relevance of education. Continuous education and training are effective in sharing knowledge and developing pain management skills [17, 18]. A recent study found that after a pain management program was introduced for nursing personnel, the number of hospitalized patients who reported moderate to severe pain as well as the psychological and physical consequences of pain decreased [17]. However, only 42.3% of nurses reported moderate to extreme satisfaction with professional pain education in critically ill patients. Satisfaction in nursing staff was not investigated in our study; however, this might be an opportunity for further research. The most common obstacles to hamper the pain assessment and management defined by nurses are as follows: sphere of nurse's activity (65.3%); patient instability (54.4%); inability to communicate with the patient (53.3%); and sedation, which hinders the assessment of pain (50%). Barriers and options for pain assessment and management along with pain training differed significantly depending on the nurses' experience and the hospital type [19].

Despite examining the data for statistically significant differences in pain monitoring between divisions across the institution, we found that statistically significant differences could not be confirmed. The study did demonstrate the percentage of documented pain recorded in the electronic medical charts by nurses varied per unit [20]. A moderately positive association was noted between work experience (in years) and the level of perceived pain intensity [12].

The research discovered the lowest values for the appropriate analgesic application in 2016. Values continued to rise in 2017 whereas a decline was noted in 2018. According to the past research, documentation of pain is poorly recorded by

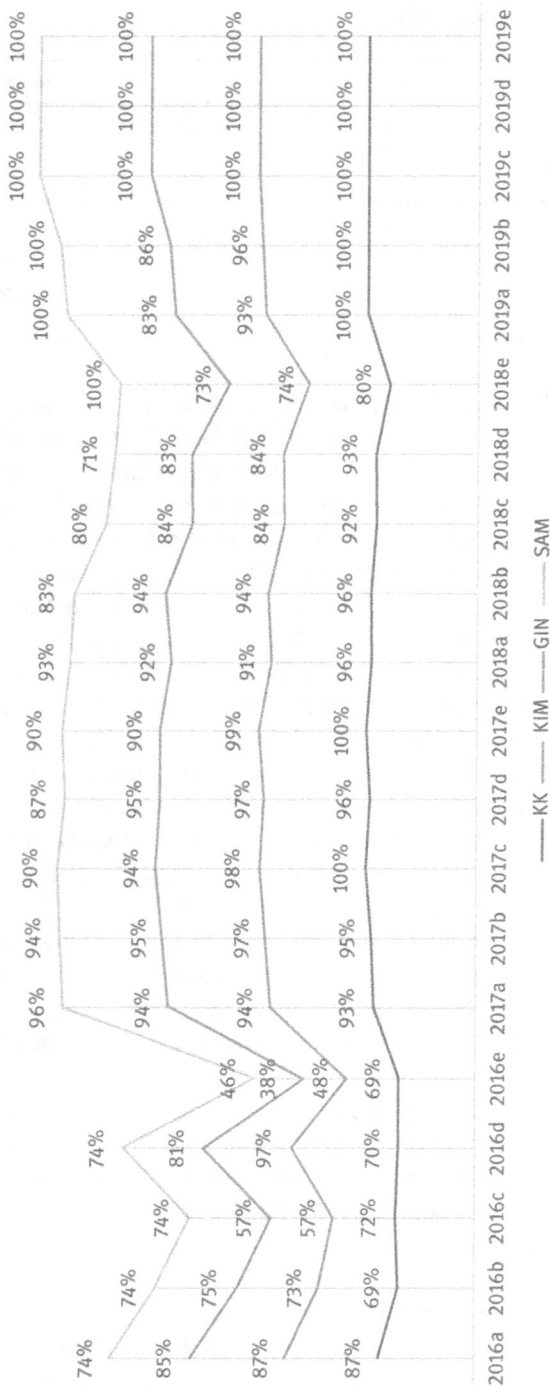

Fig. 5.1: Comparison of pain monitoring variables based on quality indicators between divisions for the period from 2016 to 2019. a, VAS at admission; b, once daily; c, before analgesics; d, appropriate analgesic administration; e, 1 h after analgesic administration; GIN, Division of Gynaecology and Obstetrics (GIN); KK, Division of Surgery; KIM, Division of Internal Medicine; SAM, increasing unevenly at independent medical departments.

nurses and even high levels of pain did not result in nurses administering more analgesics. Nurses often do not seem to trust the patient's assessment of pain [21]. Despite extensive improvements in analgesics, barriers remain in pain assessment, management, record keeping, and reassessment. Our research demonstrated that nurses would benefit from continuous training, including education on opioid use. Nurses are in a unique position for assessing and managing pain [15]. A survey investigating nurses' perspectives on barriers and options for conducting nursing assessments following workshops has identified numerous factors affecting nurses' ability to perform optimal pain assessment. The most common obstacles mentioned were lack of time, poor health, and lack of equipment [22].

Nurses' expertise and skills are essential for detecting and managing acute pain in critically ill patients [12]. In our study, the most alarming data was the following: at the beginning of monitoring in 2016, the lowest performance values across the five variables were noted in the ICUs, where critically ill patients are treated. The study highlighted the negative impact of poor cross-professional communication associated with analgesic use and the impact of nurses' workload on administering analgesics which, on the one hand, might reduce the quality and enhance the continuous pain treatment, on the other hand, in severely ill patients. It has been found that the level of pain intensity reported by nurses increased with their years of expertise. The skillset and competencies that are required for the effective and safe management of the demands posed by critically ill patients, particularly pain assessment and treatment, are very complex [11]. Inadequate acute pain management may result in higher morbidity and mortality [23, 24]. An intervention initiated by a nurse is one of the most significant strategies for managing symptoms promptly, for example, analgesia in acute pain patients. Policies or protocols for nurses, with necessary competencies adopted by the facility, usually include independent initiation of treatment based on clinical judgment and/or investigations before a physician's instructions [25]. However, in Slovenia, we have not identified such an appropriately regulated practice. A multidimensional monitoring and treatment approach is required due to the many causes of chronic pain. As a result, the quality of pain management is challenging and complex, reflecting not only decision-making in health care but also organizational structure and processes [9].

5.5 Conclusion

Quality assessment and timely intervention by nurses are critical for the management of pain and are essential for quality and evidence-based care. This study aimed to evaluate the long-term monitoring effects of pain following the introduction of a pain QI in a clinical setting in one of the tertiary institutions. Standardized tools help maintain the attention of nursing staff; however, the critical judgment of nurses is also of vital importance in the initiation of pain therapies. To identify the breadth of the issue, further research is necessary to determine whether nursing staff have sufficient education and knowledge on the importance of monitoring pain and in determining their attitudes and perceptions about pain. In-depth monitoring of pain assessment across individual units (emergency centres, ICUs, paediatric wards, and geriatric departments) and multicentre research would be reasonable. Investigation into root causes is necessary to organize further pain monitoring activities and provide support for nursing's management of pain. Better awareness of modalities aimed at pain reduction is necessary across all management levels within the facility. Furthermore, it is essential to adopt future protocols at the national level for analgesics administration.

The objectives of the research have been achieved nevertheless; the study has its limitations. This research was conducted as an analysis of pain monitoring data in a tertiary facility with the interpretation of pain monitoring over 4 years. The research results provided us an insight; however, the data cannot be generalized outside the facility due to the sample size. The fact that the produced QI is not widely accepted can also be considered a limitation to the study. Every healthcare professional is responsible for pain management and every healthcare professional should have optimal education in best practices of pain management. To ensure the generalizability of the results, we recommend that further studies be conducted with larger sample groups in all healthcare institutions in Slovenia.

References

[1] Agency for Healthcare Research and Quality. Quality indicators, 2021. (Accessed September 20, 2021, at https://www.qualityindicators.ahrq.gov)
[2] Berg K, Mor V, Morris J, Murphy KM, Moore T, Harris Y. Identification and evaluation of existing nursing homes quality indicators. HCF, 2002, 23(4), 19–36.
[3] Gajewski B, Hart S, Bergquist-Beringer S, Dunton N. Inter-rater reliability of pressure ulcer staging: Ordinal probit Bayesian hierarchical model that allows for uncertain rater response. Stat Med, 2007, 26(25), 4602–4618.
[4] Dubois CA, D'Amour D, Pomey MP, Girard F, Brault I. Conceptualizing performance of nursing care as a prerequisite for better measurement: A systematic and interpretive review. BMC Nurs, 2013, 12(7), 1–20.
[5] Mitchell PM. Definition patienty safety and quality care. In: Hughes RG, Ed. Painty safety and quality indicator: An evidence-based handbook for nurses. Agency for Healthcare Research and Quality, ZDA Rockville MD, 2008, Chapter 1.
[6] Agency for Healthcare Research and Qulaity. Improving Value and Efficiency in Hospitals and Medical Offices: A Resource List for Users of the AHRQ SOPSTM Value and Efficiency Supplemental Items, 2019. (Accessed September 20, 2021, at https://www.ahrq.gov/sites/default/files/wysiwyg/sops/quality-patient-safety/patientsafetyculture/valueresourcelist.pdf)
[7] Gregory J. Use of pain scales and observational pain assessment tools in hospital settings. RCNi, 2019, e11308.

[8]   European Pain Federation. What is the definition of pain? N.d. (Accessed September 22, 2021, https://europeanpainfederation.eu/history/what-is-pain)
[9]   De Meji N, Köke A, Thomassen I, Kallewaard JW, van Kleef M, van der Weijden T. Quality indicator fort he assessment of pain clinic care: A step forward? Quality from profesionals and patients perspective (QiPP). IASP, 2018, 12, 2593–2605.
[10]   de Meji N, Albère K, van der Weijden T, van Kleef M, Patijn J. Pain treatment facilities: Do we need quantity or quality?. J Eval Clin Pract, 2014, 20(5), 578–581.
[11]   Varndell W, Fry M, Elliott D. Pain assessment and interventions by nurses in the emergency department: A national survey. J Clin Nurs, 2020, 29(13–14), 2352–2362.
[12]   Varndell W, Fry M, Elliott D. Exploring how nurses assess, monitor and manage acute pain for adult critically ill patients in the emergency department: Protocol for a mixed methods study. Scand J Travma Resusc Emerg Med, 2017, 25(1), 75.
[13]   Casarett DJ, Hirschman BK, Miller RE, Farrar TJ. Is satisfaction with pain management a valid and reliable quality indicator for use in nursing homes? J Am Geriatr Soc, 2002, 50(12), 2029–2034.
[14]   Joy JA, Novosel LM, Ren D, Engberg S. Effect of a QI intervention on nursing assistants' pain knowledge and reporting behavior. Pain Manag Nurs, 2021, 22(2), 150–157.
[15]   Pretorius P, Searle J, Marshall B. Barriers and enablers to emergency department nurses' management of patients' pain. Pain Manag Nurs, 2015, 16(3), 372–379.
[16]   Roos-Blom MJ, Gude WT, Spijkstra JJ, de Jonge E, Dongelmans D, de Keizer NF. Measuring quality indicators to improve pain management in critically ill patients. Jcc, 2019, 49, 136–142.
[17]   Germossa GN, Hellesø R, Sjetne IS. Hospitalized patients' pain experience before and after the introduction of a nurse-based pain management programme: A separate sample pre and post study. BMC Nurs, 2019, 18(1), 40.
[18]   Sinclair PM, Kable A, Levett-Jones T, Booth D. The effectiveness of internet-based e-learning on clinician behaviour and patient outcomes: A systematic review. Ijns, 2016, 57, 70–81.
[19]   Köse Tamer L, Sucu Dağ G. The assessment of pain and the quality of postoperative pain management in surgical patients. Sage, 2020, 1–10.
[20]   Goudman L, Duarte V, De Smedt A, Copley S, Eldabe S, Moen M. Cross-country differences in pain medication before and after spinal cord stimulation: A pooled analysis of individual patient data from two prospective studies in the United Kingdom and Belgium. INS, 2021, 24.
[21]   Watt-Watson J, Stevens B, Garfinkel P, Streiner D, Gallop R. Relationship between nurses' knowledge and pain management outcomes for their postoperative cardiac patients. J Adv Nurs, 2001, 36(4), 535–545.
[22]   Baillot A, Chenail S, Barros Polita N, Simoneau M, Libourel M, Nazon E, Riesco E, Bond DS, Romain AJ. Physical activity motives, barriers, and preferences in people with obesity: A systematic review. PLoS One, 2021, 16(6), e0253114.
[23]   Lord B, Varndell W. Pain management. In: Curtis K, Ramsden C, Eds. Emergency and trauma care for nurses and paramedics. 3rd ed. Sydney, NSW, Elsevier, 2019.
[24]   Schug SA, Palmer GM, Scott DA, Halliwell R, Trinca J. Acute pain management: Scientific evidence. 4th ed, 2015.
[25]   Burgess L, Kynoch K. Effectiveness of nurse-initiated interventions on patient outcomes in the emergency department: A systematic review protocol. JBI Database System Rev Implement, 2017, 15(4), 873–881.

Lucija Gosak, Leona Cilar Budler, Amanda Briggs,
Klavdija Čuček Trifkovič, Tracy McClelland,
Nino Fijačko, Gregor Štiglic

6 Mobile phone apps' support for people with mild dementia: a systematic review

Abstract

Introduction: Dementia is a general term for various disorders characterized by loss of at least one cognitive domain. People living with mild dementia are faced with different difficulties in their daily life activities. Modern technologies, such as mobile phone apps – often called mHealth apps – can alleviate their difficulties. This paper aimed to systematically search, analyse, and synthesize mobile phone apps designed to support people living with mild dementia in daily activities in two mobile stores: Apple App and Google Play Store.

Methods: A search was conducted in May 2019 following Preferred Reporting Items for Systematic Reviews and Meta-Analyses recommendations. Results were analysed and displayed as tables and graphs. Results were synthesized using an inductive coding approach from 14 components of daily life activities for categorized nursing activities. Mobile phone apps were assessed for quality using the System Usability Scale.

Results: A total of 15 of 356 mobile phone apps were identified, applying inclusion and exclusion criteria. The inductive coding analysis identified five major themes: multi-component daily life activities, communication and feelings, recreation, eating and drinking, and movement. Most identified mobile phone apps (73%) were not mentioned in the scientific literature.

Discussion: Mobile phone apps for people living with mild dementia are mainly focused on providing information and maintaining communication skills and life activities. To a lesser extent, the apps focus on solving the problems and challenges people living with mild dementia face due to their condition.

Conclusion: Many mobile phone apps are available in the app store to support people living with mild dementia, yet only a few are focused on daily life challenges. Most of the available apps were not evaluated nor assessed for quality.

Keywords: dementia, mobile health, healthcare, everyday activities

6.1 Introduction

6.1.1 Mobile phone apps used in healthcare

In the past decade, many improvements in technology have been made. Especially, improvements are visible in using mobile phone devices, nowadays called smartphones. Smartphone ownership is growing globally; it is estimated that more than 5 billion people own mobile devices, with more than half of these connections being smartphones [1]. Due to this vast growth in ownership, stakeholders in this industry are capitalizing by building mobile phone software applications (apps) for various uses. Advancement has led to many apps being developed available in social media, games, aid shopping or travel, and so on [2]. Depending on the operating system (OS), different platforms are available, which enable the use of the apps. A mobile OS is a software platform where apps run on mobile devices. Companies dominating the mobile OSs market are Apple Store with iOS and Google Play with Android OS [3, 4].

While the first apps initiated were for organizational and later recreational use [5], many apps have since been developed for use in healthcare, both for professionals and patients. Apps in the healthcare field are gaining high popularity in recent years [6, 7]. These apps are specialized for conditions including diabetes management, alleviating gastrointestinal problems, HIV/AIDS treatments, assisting with learning difficulties, promoting mental health and women's health [2, 8]. Mobile health (mHealth) has shown improvements in the quality, access to, and delivery in terms of sourcing health information, accessing services and skilled help, and promoting positive changes in health-related behaviours to prevent the onset of acute and chronic diseases [9].

6.1.2 Challenges of mild dementia

Dementia is a chronic condition that is associated with ageing. Consequences are evident for patients, significant others, and healthcare systems [10]. Dementia is a term for various disorders characterized by memory impairment and at least one other cognitive domain (executive function, aphasia, apraxia, and agnosia). There are numerous subtypes of dementia, including Alzheimer's disease and frontotemporal lobar dementia [11]. Different stages of dementia bring different challenges. Mild dementia is recognized as a cognitive impairment that represents the potential to grow into serious types of dementia. Patients with mild dementia are independent in simpler activities of daily living (ADLs) [12]. The number of people living with mild dementia continues to grow globally [13]. Thus, many studies focus on dementia prevention [14, 15], treatment, and healthcare [16]. Few focus on helping people living with mild dementia in their ADLs. Virginia Henderson [17] was the first theorist that focused on ADLs and categorized nursing activities into 14 components based on human needs.

6.1.3 Prior work in the field of dementia and technology use

Dementia affects people with mild dementia and their families, has a significant impact on their lives and health outcomes, and presents a daily challenge [18]. One of the most challenging symptoms of dementia is losing the ability to live independently. Thus, many patients struggle with basic ADLs, including movement, dressing, recreation, communication, eating, and drinking. ADLs such as recreation and movement are usually neglected yet important in maintaining the quality of life [19]. Apps can provide adequate support for people living with mild dementia in their ADLs [20], encouraging their independence, but available apps show limited functions [21]. There are many apps available for people with severe types of dementia. However, little is known about their usability and health outcomes [22].

The app industry is growing rapidly, and new apps are available almost daily. As these apps saturate the market, there is a need to evaluate these apps in usability and content. The review aims to identify and evaluate apps available to support people living with mild dementia throughout their daily lives, specifically with their ADLs. People living with mild dementia are still living in a community setting, and mobile apps help them to manage ADLs independently and are important in this respect to improve their quality of life and relieve the burden on healthcare staff.

6.2 Methods

6.2.1 Design

A systematic review, analysis, and synthesis of apps for mild dementia were conducted. The steps of the review were: (1) app review through an initial screening of all retrieved apps; (2) review of the included apps; (3) data extraction; (4) data analysis; and (5) data synthesis [23].

6.2.2 Search strategy

The search for apps was done in May 2019 using inclusion and exclusion criteria. A search was performed in iOS OS in iPhone (12.3.1 software version) and Android in Samsung S8 (Pie 9.0 software version). Apps that were developed for helping people living with mild dementia were included. Moreover, we included apps available in mobile stores in Slovenia and the English language.

6.2.3 App selection process

The review process was followed by Preferred Reporting Items for Systematic Reviews and Meta-analyses – PRISMA recommendation [24]. A search was conducted by a researcher (LC) in App Store (for iOS) and Google Play Store (for Android) using the keyword "dementia". Next, the names of mobile phones from each store were transferred into a Microsoft Excel spreadsheet for duplication removal. Two independent researchers (LG and NF) have reviewed the titles and icons of mobile apps in the Google Play Store, and two independent researchers (LC and GS) have reviewed the titles and icons of mobile apps in the App Store. This approach has been used previously in similar papers [25, 26]. A discussion between members of the research team resolved inconsistencies in the review of apps. Moreover, apps were reviewed by the full description, which included a review of the information about the app characteristics, written information, pictures, and videos. We also investigated if apps were mentioned in scientific literature. In the final phase, we excluded paid apps, as we wanted to include in the final analysis only those apps that are accessible to all users. We have also excluded apps that only targeted specific groups and not people living with mild dementia. We also excluded apps that were only for learning.

6.2.4 Data exclusion

Apps that did not fit the inclusion criteria in App Store were excluded. Apps were excluded if they were games, not adapted for people living with mild dementia, in different languages, commercial, designed for practitioners and caregivers, testing and screening tools, and other apps not relevant to dementia. Moreover, in the full review of installed apps, the exclusion criteria included ADL – learning (information, diaries, orientation, reminders) and only general information about dementia.

6.2.5 Data synthesis

Data were synthesized using mapping coding approach [27] steps in a systematic review of articles. Five major themes were used for mapping codes: multi-ADL, communication and emotions, recreation, eating and drinking, and movement, conducted from 14 components of ADLs [17].

6.2.6 Quality assessment

App quality was assessed using System Usability Scale (SUS) [28], which has been previously used in a similar paper relating to app reviews [29]. The result of SUS was obtained by calculating the score contribution from each item. Each item ranged from 0 to 4 for items 1, 3, 5, 7, and 9 and from 4 to 0 for items 2, 4, 6, 8, and 10. The overall value was obtained by multiplying the score by 2.5.

6.3 Results

6.3.1 General characteristics of included apps

There were 448 apps identified in both App Stores. After removing 92 duplicates, apps were reviewed by name and icon, with 69 apps remaining for review by description. Using the PRISMA recommendations [24] and inclusion and exclusion criteria, 15 apps (4.21% of all identified) were extracted and analysed (Fig. 6.1).

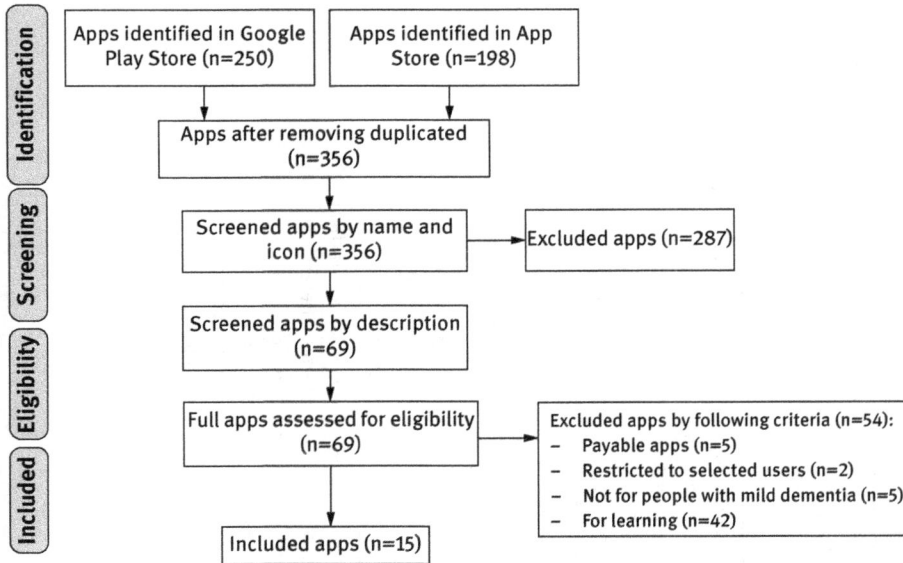

Fig. 6.1: PRISMA flow chart.

Table 6.1 presents the main characteristics of 15 included apps (app name, platform, price, version, category, scientific based-literature, developer, and rating). One app was payable, but the trial version was available. We used information from the Apple App Store for apps that were available on both platforms.

Tab. 6.1: Characteristics of included apps.

Apps name	Target group and target disease	Short description	Operating system	Developer	Version	Category	Price	Mentioned in the scientific literature	Rating (0–5)	SUS
9zest Parkinson's Therapy	The app is primarily aimed at Parkinson's patients and anyone who needs help with eating, drinking, dressing, and other daily activities	App helps users with everyday activities such as eating, drinking, writing, dressing, and walking	iOS, Android OS	9zest, Inc	3.2.0	Medical	$11.49 monthly plan	Yes	4.5	95
Activities for care: elderly dementia LD seniors	Elderly people with dementia LD	App allows you to monitor patients' electronic vital records from images to videos	iOS, Android OS	RemindMecare	1.0.1	Medical	Free of charge	No	4.8	75
Alzheimer's Daily Companion	For family carers of patients with Alzheimer's disease or other forms of dementia	App includes practical tips for different situations that dementia patients or their carers face on a daily basis	iOS, Android OS	Home Instead, Inc.	2.0.4	Lifestyle	Free of charge	Yes	4.4	85

Talk Around It USA Free	It is aimed at people with word-finding difficulties and has been used to treat conditions such as aphasia, anomia, stroke, dementia, Alzheimer's disease, and autism	App helps with speech and language problems	iOS, Android OS	Neuro Hero Ltd	2.01	Medical	Free of charge	No	Not enough ratings	72.5
Brain Injury – One Skill Videos	For patients with brain injuries	App includes a variety of videos for patients	Android OS	Neuro Hero Ltd	1.0	Medical	Free of charge	No	3.8	72.5
LookBack VR	For people with dementia	App includes VR to stimulate reminiscence and encourage techniques for making contact and improving well-being	iOS, Android OS	VRTU Inc	1.2	Health and fitness	Free of charge	Yes	5.0	57.5
DemKonnect – Dementia Care App	For dementia care providers	App provides access to care, contact with a professional, and access to useful information	iOS, Android OS	Nightingales Medical Trust	1.0.12	Health and fitness	Free of charge	No	Not enough ratings	90

(continued)

Tab. 6.1 (continued)

Apps name	Target group and target disease	Short description	Operating system	Developer	Version	Category	Price	Mentioned in the scientific literature	Rating (0–5)	SUS
Dementia – Cuomo	For dementia patients	App encourages social activity and communication between patients, carers, and healthcare professionals	iOS	Cuomo Limited	1.02	Social networking	Free of charge	No	Not enough ratings	90
Memory Helper Carer Assistance	For carers of people living with memory loss, Alzheimer's disease, or dementia	App facilitates communication with family, carers, and provides useful reminders	iOS, Android OS	Judy Handel	1.3	Medical	Free of charges	No	5.0	77.5
Approach Staffordshire	Patients with memory loss	App includes various reminders, news, and questionnaires for the patient	iOS, Android OS	More IT Ltd.	6.99	Education	Free of charges	No	Not enough ratings	77.5

App	Target group	Description	OS	Developer	Version	Category	Price		Rating	SUS
LifeVU	For the elderly and lonely	App makes it easier to communicate with family and friends who are lonely by allowing you to send pictures, messages, and posts	Android OS	LifeVU	2.0	Social networking	Free of charges	No	5.0	70
Care and Connect	For doctors, patients, and their families	App enables communication between members of the healthcare team and users of the healthcare service	Android OS, iOS	Newcastle University	1.2	Lifestyle	Free of charge	Yes	Not enough ratings	85
AidEye	For the visually impaired, dyslexic, demented, elderly, and all visually impaired	App identifies objects and provides users with an audio description of the identified object	Android OS	Gocube Technology	1.0.7	Lifestyle	Free of charge	No	Not enough ratings	72.5
MIND Diet Plan	To reduce the risk of Alzheimer's disease and weight loss	App encourages healthy eating to slow the loss of brain function	Android OS	Axcore	1.1	Health and fitness	Free of charge	No	5.0	80
MyAreas	For all persons, primarily those with memory impairment	App is a safety net for people in case they get lost outside their homes	iOS	Applicate IT ApS	1.4.1	Utilities	Free of charge	No	Not enough ratings	85

SUS, System Usability Scale.

Most (n = 9; 60%) of the identified apps were available for both OSs (iOS and Android). Four (26.66%) apps were available only on Android OS and two (13.33%) on iOS. Apps were categorized in both OS as follows: social networking (n = 2), medical (n = 5), education (n = 1), utilities (n = 1), lifestyle (n = 3), or health and fitness (n = 3). Only four apps (9zest Parkinson's Therapy, Alzheimer's Daily Companion, LookBack VR, and Care and Connect) were mentioned in the scientific literature. The highest SUS score was 95 (9zest Parkinson's Therapy), and the lowest was 57.5 (LookBack VR). None of the analysed apps scored 0 (minimum) or 100 (maximum).

6.3.2 Synthesis

The data synthesis followed the steps of mapping coding. Five major themes were used for mapping codes: multi-ADL, communication and emotions, recreation, eating and drinking, and movement, conducted from 14 components of ADLs [17] (Tab. 6.2).

Tab. 6.2: Mobile apps are categorized by components of ADLs – the synthesis.

MA	Free codes	Subcategory	Main category
1	Balance and posture, eating and drinking, speech, reducing falls, dressing	Multicomponent	Multi-ADL
2	Personal profile, photos, videos, music conversation recording, activity creation tool, family engagement, calendars, alerts, home Integration, hydration alerts, monitoring		
3	Tips and practical advice for all behaviours and situations they face daily		
4	Word retrieval, speech, and language techniques	Communicate with others	Communication and emotions
5	Words, speech, language		
6	Help connect	Connect with others	
7	Communication, support		
8	Community, support, friendships, expressing feelings	Expressing emotions, needs, fears, or opinions	
9	Communication tool, information, reminders, notes		
10	Communication, messages		
11	Sending meaningful messages, pics, and posts enhances social interactions		

Tab. 6.2 (continued)

MA	Free codes	Subcategory	Main category
12	Outside recreation, communities, places, wayfinding	Play or participate in various forms of recreation	Recreation
13	Integration, independence, restaurants, home, calmness, wayfinding, friendly places		
14	Diet, lower blood pressure, reduce risk of diseases, eating barriers, fruit consumption, BMI	Eat and drink adequately	Eating and drinking
15	Movement, move outside home	Maintain desirable postures	Movement

MA, mobile app.

The outcomes of identified apps were heterogenic; thus, further analysis was impossible.

Five main categories and seven sub-categories were identified in the mobile apps. The ADL category referred to multi-components emphasizing breast profile, videos, falls, etc. The Communication and emotions category included three sub-categories referring to communicating with others, connecting with others and expressing emotions. There were also categories relating to exercise, recreation, drinking, and eating.

Three apps (20%) were identified that included more than one category of ADLs (9zest Parkinson's Therapy, Activities for care: elderly dementia LD seniors and Alzheimer's Daily Companion). Most of the identified apps ($n = 8$) focused on communication and expressing feelings. Moreover, two apps focused on recreation: one on eating and drinking and one on movement.

6.4 Discussion

Involvement in the daily activities of people with mild dementia significantly influences their quality of life and overall well-being [30]. However, there is limited research to investigate how to ensure their involvement in ADLs. Five main themes were identified through systematic review, analysis, and synthesis of apps for people living with mild dementia: multi-components; communication and feelings; recreation; eating and drinking; and movement.

People living with mild dementia are often excluded from social activities due to memory loss, loss of confidence, negative reactions from other people, or understanding issues. Possible solutions are dismantling external barriers to participation in society and enabling people living with mild dementia to participate in social life in a meaningful way [31]. Giebel et al. [19] found that impairments related to social activities caused by dementia significantly affect people's well-being with dementia. Moreover, people living with mild dementia pointed out that one of the most meaningful activities in daily life is being connected with self, others, and the environment [32]. Communication and feelings apps focus on speech and language, word retrieval (Talk Around It USA Free), support, friendship, expressing feelings, sending messages, and enhancing social interactions (Brain Injury – One Skill Videos, LookBack VR, and DemKonnect – Dementia Care App). Identified apps support people living with mild dementia to stay active and connect with significant others (e.g. writing with peers). DemKonnect – Dementia Care App also allows video calls, but only with an expert.

Therapeutic recreation has a positive impact on people living with mild dementia in terms of behaviour and well-being [33]. The study conducted in 2016 among Chinese older people living with mild dementia, showed potential improvement in cognitive function, daily living ability, and behavioural and psychological symptoms after implementing a program based on recreation. Interventions included art activities, games, and music activities [34]. Promising results were demonstrated using an interpersonal program for people with dementia, indicating significant correlations between engagement types, behavioural outcomes, and quality of life of people living with mild dementia [35]. This review yielded the following codes associated with recreation in people living with mild dementia: places; communities; integration; independence; restaurants; home; calmness; wayfinding; and friendly places (Care and Connect, and AidEye).

The risk of dehydration and malnutrition in people living with mild dementia is higher than in healthy older people. People living with mild dementia often have difficulties with their eating and drinking habits. This may occur due to their memory loss, resulting in, amongst other things, forgetting about eating and drinking, problems with swallowing, institutionalization, lack of caregivers, and lack of time. Hooper [36] found in their study that people with dementia are often dehydrated. Bunn et al. [37] concluded that this could be decreased if people living with mild dementia eat meals with caregivers, has family-style meals, soothing mealtime music, constant access to snacks, and has longer mealtimes and constant support from caregivers. This cannot always be established; thus, mobile phone apps show significant opportunities with alarms and reminders. Identified apps have the following features linked to eating and drinking: diet, BMI measurements, and fruit consumption (MIND Diet Plan).

People living with mild dementia may be frequently inactive, influencing their mood, social interaction, and overall health. Tobiasson et al. [38] found that physical activity in people living with mild dementia increases satisfaction with life and has positive health outcomes. Going out of the house may be challenging for people with memory loss; thus, apps with an integrated Global Positioning System – GPS may potentially support people living with mild dementia and their caregivers.

Only one app was identified that supports people living with mild dementia in their daily movements – MyAreas. This app encourages a person living with mild dementia to move around and not get lost. It is available only for iOS OS.

6.4.1 Limitations of the review

A possible limitation in this systematic review of apps for people with mild dementia is that not all OSs were included in the search. Dementia is a term used for various symptoms and stages of memory impairment, and people with long-term dementia may not be able to use a mobile phone or mobile phone apps. Moreover, mobile phone apps were evaluated by researchers included in the study and not by people with mild dementia; thus, the app's estimated usability might be biased. Outcome measures used supported in ADLs for people living with mild dementia. Mobile phone apps showed various results (heterogeneity); thus, any further analysis or synthesis was not conducted.

6.5 Conclusion

Mobile phone apps can provide adequate support for people with mild-to-moderate dementia in ADLs. Many available phone apps focus on giving information about dementia; fewer are available to support them in ADLs. The most valuable apps compose more ADLs (9zest Parkinson's Therapy, Activities for care: elderly dementia LD seniors, and Alzheimer's Daily Companion) because it is easier to have one app for multiple activities, especially for those targeting individuals with memory loss problems. The research does not well support mobile phone apps in connection to dementia and ADLs. Moreover, there is no sufficient evidence or quality appraisal tools for evaluating mobile phone apps that would allow us to recommend quality apps for older people living with mild dementia.

References

[1] Taylor K, Silver L. Smartphone ownership is growing rapidly around the world, but not always equally, 2019. (Accessed May 15, 2019, at https://www.pewglobal.org/2019/02/05/smart phone-ownership-is-growing-rapidly-around-the-world-but-not-always-equally/).
[2] Hanrahan C, Augngst TD, Cole S. Evaluating mobile medical applications. Bethesda, American Society of Health-System Pharmacists, 2014.
[3] Okediran OO. Mobile operating systems and application development platforms: A survey. Int J Adv Networking Appl, 2014, 6(1), 2195–2201.

[4]   Hannover Medical School. Chances and Risks of Mobile Health Apps (CHARISMHA), 2016. (Accessed February 2, 2019, at https://www.bundesgesundheitsministerium.de/fileadmin/ Dateien/3_Downloads/A/App-Studie/charismha_abr_v.01.1e-20160606.pdf).

[5]   Malizia A, Olsen KA. Has everything been invented? on software development and the future of apps. Computer, 2011, 44(9), 112–111.

[6]   AppBrain. Android statistics, 2018. (Accessed May 30, 2019, at http://www.appbrain.com/ stats/android-market-app-categories).

[7]   Pocketgamer.biz. App store metrics, 2018. (Accessed May 30, 2019, at http://www.pocket gamer.biz/metrics/app-store/).

[8]   Deep Knowledge Ventures. Mobile Tech Mobile Apps: Landscape Overview. 2017. (Accessed February 19, 2019 at http://analytics.dkv.global/data/pdf/Health-Tech-Mobile-Apps-Analytical-Report.pdf).

[9]   WHO. mHealth: Use of appropriate digital technologies for public health. Geneva, WHO, 2018.

[10]   Borda MG, Soennesyn H, Steves CJ, Vik-Mo AO, Pérez-Zepeda MU, Aarsland D. Frailty in older adults with mild dementia: Dementia with lewy bodies and Alzheimer's disease. Dement Geriatr Cogn Disord Extra, 2019, 9(1), 176–183.

[11]   Volos LI. Vascular dementia: Qualitative analysis of the angioarchitectonics of the cerebral cortex 2022.

[12]   Knopman DS, Petersen RC. Mild cognitive impairment and mild dementia: A clinical perspective. Mayo Clin Proc, 2014, 89(10), 1452–1459.

[13]   Powell T. Health policy and dementia. Curr Psychiatry Rep, 2018, 20(1), 1–5.

[14]   Kenigsberg PA, Aquino JP, Berard A, Gzil F, Andrieu S, Banerjee S, Bremond F, Buee L, Cohen-Mansfield J, Mangialasche F, Platel H. Dementia beyond 2025: Knowledge and uncertainties. Dementia, 2016, 15(1), 6–21.

[15]   Livingston G, Sommerlad A, Orgeta V, Costafreda SG, Huntley J, Ames D, Ballard C, Banerjee S, Burns A, Cohen-Mansfield J, Cooper C. Dementia prevention, intervention, and care. Lancet, 2017, 390(10113), 2673–2734.

[16]   Schmidt H, Eisenmann Y, Golla H, Voltz R, Perrar KM. Needs of people with advanced dementia in their final phase of life: A multi-perspective qualitative study in nursing homes. Palliat Med, 2018, 32(3), 657–667.

[17]   Henderson V, Nite G. Principles and practice of nursing. 6th ed. London, International Council of Nurses, 1978.

[18]   Nehen HG, Hermann DM. Supporting dementia patients and their caregivers in daily life challenges: Review of physical, cognitive and psychosocial intervention studies. Eur J Neurol, 2015, 22(2), 246–e20.

[19]   Giebel CM, Challis DJ, Montaldi D. A revised interview for deterioration in daily living activities in dementia reveals the relationship between social activities and well-being. Dementia, 2016, 15(5), 1068–1081.

[20]   Klimova B, Bouckova Z, Toman J. Mobile phone apps as support tools for people with dementia. In: Advanced multimedia and ubiquitous engineering, 2018, 7–12.

[21]   Brown EL, Ruggiano N, Li J, Clarke PJ, Kay ES, Hristidis V. Smartphone-based health technologies for dementia care: Opportunities, challenges, and current practices. J Appl Gerontol, 2019, 38(1), 73–91.

[22]   Bateman DR, Srinivas B, Emmett TW, Schleyer TK, Holden RJ, Hendrie HC, Callahan CM. Categorising health outcomes and efficacy of mHealth apps for persons with cognitive impairment: A systematic review. J Med Internet Res, 2017, 19(8), e7814.

[23]   Khan KS, Kunz R, Kleinen J, Antes G. Five steps to conducting a systematic review. J R Soc Med, 2003, 96(3), 11–121.

[24] Moher D, Liberati A, Tetzlaff J, Altman DG, PRISMA Group*. Preferred reporting items for systematic reviews and meta-analyses: The PRISMA statement. Ann Intern Med, 2009, 151(4), 264–269.

[25] Fijacko N, Brzan PP, Stiglic G. Mobile applications for type 2 diabetes risk estimation: A systematic review. J Med Syst, 2015, 39(124), 1–10.

[26] Furlong LM, Morris ME, Erickson S, Serry TA. Quality of mobile phone and tablet mobile apps for speech sound disorders: Protocol for an evidence-based appraisal. JMIR Res Protoc, 2016, 5(4), e233.

[27] Locock L, Graham C, King J, Parkin S, Chisholm A, Montgomery C, Gibbons E, Ainley E, Bostock J, Gager M, Churchill N. Understanding how front-line staff use patient experience data for service improvement: An exploratory case study evaluation. Health Serv Delivery Res, 2020, 8(13).

[28] Brooke J. SUS: A 'quick and dirty' usability scale. In: Jordan PW, Thomas B, Weerdmeester BA, McClelland IL, eds. Usability evaluation in industry. London, Taylor and Francis, 1996, 189–194.

[29] Ahn C, Cho Y, Oh J, Song Y, Lim TH, Kang H, Lee J. Evaluation of smartphone applications for cardiopulmonary resuscitation training in South Korea. BioMed Res Int, 2016, 1, 6418710.

[30] Smith D, de Lange J, Willemse B, Twisk J, Pot AM. Activity involvement and quality of life of people at different stages of dementia in long term care facilities. Aging Ment Health, 2015, 20(1), 100–109.

[31] Clare L. Rehabilitation for people living with dementia: A practical framework of positive support. PLoS Med, 2017, 14(3), 1–4.

[32] Han A, Radel J, McDowd JM, Sabata D. Perspectives of people with dementia about meaningful activities: A Synthesis. Am J Alzheimers Dis Other Demen, 2016, 31(2), 115–123.

[33] Cohen-Mansfield J, Hirshfeld K, Gavendo R, Corey E, Hai T. Activity-in-a-box for engaging persons with dementia in groups: Implications for therapeutic recreation practice. Am J Recreat Ther, 2016, 15(3), 70–83.

[34] Li D, Li X. The effect of folk recreation program in improving symptoms: A study of Chinese elder dementia patients. Int J Geriatr Psychiatry, 2016, 32(8), 901–908.

[35] Janke MC, Purnell I, Watts C, Shores K. Associations between engagement types, outcome behaviors, and quality of life for adults with dementia participating in intergenerational programs. Ther Recreat J, 2019, 53(2), 132–148.

[36] Hooper L. Why, oh why, are so many older adults not drinking enough fluid? J Acad Nutr Diet, 2016, 116(5), 774–778.

[37] Bunn DK, Abdelhamid A, Copley M, Cowap V, Dickinson A, Howe A, Killett A, Poland F, Potter JF, Richardson K, Smithard D. Effectiveness of interventions to indirectly support food and drink intake in people with dementia: Eating and drinking well IN dementiA (EDWINA) systematic review. BMC Geriatr, 2016, 16(1), 1–21.

[38] Tobiasson H, Sundblad Y, Walldius Å, Hedman A. Designing for active life: Moving and being moved together with dementia patients. Int J Des, 2015, 9(3), 47–62.

Zvonka Fekonja, Sergej Kmetec, Urška Fekonja,
Nataša Mlinar Reljić, Irma Mikkonen, Barbara Donik

7 Ethical issues in palliative care and end-of-life care experienced by nursing staff within nursing homes: a cross-sectional study

Abstract

Background: Globally, the proportion of older people is increasing along with life expectancy. A significant proportion of older people spend their terminal phase of life in a nursing home, where palliative care is important. This study aims to determine the type and frequency of ethical issues among the nurses delivering palliative care in nursing homes.

Method: A cross-sectional survey method was used. Data were collected using a survey questionnaire. One hundred and eighteen nurses in two nursing homes in Slovenia completed the questionnaire. The instrument explored the frequency of ethical issues in nursing homes while providing palliative care to older dying people.

Results: The survey showed that the healthcare teams enjoy caring for dying older people; they feel qualified to perform palliative care, which is crucial for ensuring the comfort of the dying person. The survey results show that frequent ethical issues arise in professional, practice, and relational issues.

Conclusion: The comparative surveys showed similar results; we have concluded that palliative care in institutional care is still not well organised or supported by continuous training for nurses.

Keywords: aged, nurses, palliative care, nursing home

7.1 Introduction

Globally, the proportion of older people in the population is increasing rapidly. However, increasing life expectancy increases the chance of developing chronically non-communicable diseases in individuals [1]. A significant proportion of older people, most of whom require complex terminal medical care [2], die in nursing homes. In Europe, between 12% and 38% of older people die in a nursing home, and this is expected to increase in the future [3]. The ageing trend will continue and put increased pressure on resources in care homes due to the increased prevalence of chronic diseases and complex comorbidities [4]. In doing so, healthcare professionals need to pay attention to older people's physical, psychological, social, and spiritual needs to meet and provide holistic palliative care [5] in the process of caring for a dying an older person.

The concept of palliative care is closely related to the terminal phase of life. Its goal is to provide older people in the terminal phase of the disease with a better quality of life and relief from symptoms and the disease's consequences [6]. Palliative care during the dying period is essential to provide older people with all physical, emotional, and spiritual needs. The goal of palliative care is not only focused on quality of life but also on dignified death [7]. Nursing staff in nursing homes are often exposed to the deaths of their residents; with respectful professional and understanding treatment, they contribute daily to the dignity of older people dying in nursing homes [8]. An ethical approach to the care of older people plays an important role in palliative care, which is important in the process of dying, as it preserves dignity. Ethical issues in palliative care often stem from concerns about the adequacy of care and what older people need [2]. Ethical issues or challenges appear more often when there is disagreement, uncertainty, or doubts about making morally good or correct decisions [6]. In palliative care, ethical issues arise more often in advanced care planning, inadequate management of distressing symptoms, involvement or support of the care partners, and at the end of life care [9]. Ethical issues often have harmful consequences for the individual nurse in the form of moral distress, burnout and, as a result, a change of profession [10]. Many studies have found that the problem in nursing homes is a lack of experienced staff and materials, time, knowledge, and an ethical approach to providing quality holistic palliative care to dying older people, in their last days [4, 9]. Abudari and Zahreddine [11] conclude that palliative care should be introduced in nursing school systems worldwide, as they found that nurses do not have sufficient knowledge and experience to be able to provide palliative care independently.

Similarly, Leclerc and Lessard [12] showed significant differences in knowledge, handling, communication, and working with the dying in the nursing home among the staff; none had received specific training in palliative care. Furthermore, Simon, Ramsenthaler [13], and Kmetec and Fekonja [4] found that a person-centred approach is important to people in palliative care. Health professionals, who most often provide nursing care to older people needing palliative care, experience more ethical problems [14], so this chapter aims to determine the type and frequency of ethical issues among the nurses, during the delivery of palliative care in nursing homes.

7.2 Methods

7.2.1 Study design

The study uses quantitative research methodology, a deductive approach within the positivist paradigm characterizing such a methodology [15]. This paradigm provides us with an overview of ethical issues related to dying older people in nursing homes, from the perspective of the nursing team and their perspective on palliative care. A cross-sectional survey using a questionnaire was used. To ensure the reliability and rigour of the study and reporting results, we followed the STROBE guidelines [16].

7.2.2 Settings and participants

The settings were two nursing homes in Slovenia. Convenience sampling was used, and employees who were on the morning shift on a given day were involved [15]. We involved all members of the nursing care team, who work in nursing homes and have experience providing palliative care to dying older people; 118 members of the nursing care team participated in the study by completing the survey anonymously and voluntarily. Individuals were included in the study if they were >18 years of age, provided palliative care to older people, and worked in a nursing care team. Participants were included based on the eligibility criteria; they were working in a nursing home at the time of data collecting and had provided informed consent. We collected the data between December 2019 and May 2020.

7.2.3 Data collection and measures

The questionnaire *Ethical Issues and Palliative Care for Nursing Homes* (EPiCNH) by Preshaw et al. [10] was used and was designed to analyse ethical issues regarding palliative care in a nursing home. Before using the research instrument, permission from the original author was obtained. The questionnaire consists of two parts. In the first part, the questions refer to the demographic characteristics of the respondents. In the second part, in 26 statements, the respondents indicated the occurrence of ethical situations in three areas: professional issues/issues in practice, organisational issues, and relational issues. Participants had to rate each statement from 0 ("did not occur") to 4 ("high frequency of occurrence").

Respondents were verbally informed in advance about the survey and were guaranteed anonymity and the freedom to choose to take part in the survey. The content validity of the questionnaire was guided by Polit and Beck's [15] guidelines. We also checked the appropriateness of the questionnaire structure, appearance, feasibility, readability, consistency of style between questions, formatting, and clarity of language. Ten experts were purposively chosen for their knowledge of palliative care and heart failure. The expert panel subsequently approved the questionnaire. The questionnaire was pilot-tested with a small sample of the nursing care team ($n = 67$) to assess its reliability using Cronbach's alpha. The Cronbach's alpha of the questionnaire was 0.92.

Of the 118 eligible participants, 36 professional caregivers, 62 nursing assistants, and 20 registered nurses agreed to participate in the study and completed the questionnaires (response rate = 69%). As all the questions required mandatory answers, there were no missing values in any of the variables for data collected.

7.2.4 Data analysis

Data (anonymized) were entered and managed using IBM SPSS version 28 and a database was created for further analysis. Descriptive statistics were displayed as numbers on total (percentage), mean (M), and standard deviation (SD).

7.2.5 Ethical approval

Before the study, approval was obtained from the competent ethics committee in Slovenia (ref. no.: 038/2018/2510-2/504). Study participants were informed about the purpose and objectives of the study, confidentiality, anonymity, and voluntariness. Participation could be terminated at any time before submitting the completed questionnaire. Participants were allowed to see the results of the study, if they wished. The study strictly adhered to the ethical principles of the Declaration of Helsinki [17] and the provisions of the Oviedo Convention [18].

7.3 Results

7.3.1 Participants

Of the 118 respondents, 88.9% ($n = 87$) were women and many participants, 53% ($n = 62$), had a secondary level of education – nursing assistants, 31% ($n = 36$) were carers, and 16% ($n = 20$) were Registered Nurses. The mean age of participants was 39 (SD = 11.52) years. The oldest respondent was 60 years old, and the youngest was 19. The mean length of work experience of all participants in the survey was 17 (SD = 0.78) years, with the longest being 40 years and the shortest, three months. The mean length of work experience in the current job was 11 (SD = 9.06) years, with a minimum of three months and a maximum of 38 years (Tab. 7.1).

Almost half of the respondents, 48% ($n = 57$), see a dying person at work often, which means at least once a month, and 35% ($n = 30$) very often, at least twice a month. Only 0.8% ($n = 1$) of the respondents had never met a dying older person, and 21.2% ($n = 25$) had rarely met them. We wanted to know how the nursing care team felt about working with dying older people: 62.7% ($n = 74$) are empathetic and think about it at home; 27.1% ($n = 32$) consider nursing as their job and have no special feelings; and 10.2% ($n = 12$) are more sympathetic to the dying person compared to other employees. The care of the dying is very important, with 113% ($n = 95.7$) of respondents agreeing and 4.2% ($n = 5$) disagreeing (Tab. 7.1).

Tab. 7.1: Demographic characteristics of included nurses.

Variables ($n = 118$)		%(n)		
Gender				
Male		11.1(13)		
Female		88.9(105)		
Education				
Professional caregivers		31(36)		
Nursing assistants		53(62)		
Registered nurse		16(20)		
Frequency of encounters with the dying:				
I have never met before		0.8(1)		
Rare (up to twice a year)		21.2(25)		
Often (at least once a month)		48(57)		
Very common (more than twice a month)		30(35)		
Feelings when working with the dying:				
I have no special emotions		27.1(32)		
I feel empathetic, and I think about it at home too		62.7(74)		
I am more in favour of the person than others		10.2(12)		
The importance of caring for the elderly in the process of dying:				
Yes		95.7(113)		
No		4.2(5)		
	M(SD)		Min	Max
Age	39(11.52)		19	60
Total years of work experience	17(0.78)		0	40
Work experience in a nursing home	11(9.06)		0	38

M, mean; min, minimum; max, maximum; *n*, sample size; SD, standard deviation; %, per cent of participants.

7.3.2 Ethical issues

The survey showed that ethical issues often occur in different areas of providing palliative care in nursing homes. In professional issues/problems in practice and relationships, difficulties often arise concerning making decisions in the older person's best interests, to avoid unnecessary harm (M = 3.09; SD = 0.99) (Tab. 7.2). The fear of death is not a particular problem for the respondents, as 62.7% (n = 74) do not avoid the dying person due to fear of death. Very often, in 14% (n = 11.9), the subject of the death of older people is deliberately avoided. Fifty-six per cent (n = 56) of respondents strongly agreed that the nursing care team is key to ensuring the comfort of the dying older person. When a person is dying, the time of treatment is crucial. This is confirmed by the analysis of the statement, where 46% (n = 46) of the respondents strongly agree with this statement, 41% (n = 41) agree, and 9% (n = 9) cannot decide. Only 4% (n = 4) disagreed or strongly disagreed with the statement, meaning that the time of dealing with the dying person is unimportant to them.

Considering the family's wishes for care as opposed to their own opinion was the second most chosen statement (M = 2.77; SD = 0.85) related to attention to residents' care needs. The older people's rejection of food and liquids was the third most commonly endorsed statement (M = 2.72; SD = 1.08), and the fourth most widely reported statement was witnessing distress by family members or care partners (M = 2, 60; SD = 1.20). The fifth most frequently reported point was poor communication with staff, resulting in more inferior quality of care (M = 2.05; SD = 1.06). These survey ratings highlight ethical issues in relationships as the most common of these topics.

Organisational ethical issues, particularly lack of resources, were reported to occur frequently in practice by respondents, such as lack of time for providing older people with needed nursing care (M = 2.48; SD = 0.98), lack of physician support for older people nursing care (M = 2.20; SD = 1.21) and involvement in non-care activities, which reduce the time spent with the older people (M = 2.14; SD = 1.21). These items were scored infrequently on the frequency score, with mean scores ranging from 0.81 to 2.48. We noticed that the nursing team's lack of resources within the nursing home does not pose a major problem in providing sufficient palliative nursing care for the dying person, as 48.3% (n = 57) never or rarely have problems with this. Of the participants, 27% (n = 32) said they often experience a lack of resources, while 24.6% (n = 29) said it happens.

Regarding competence to provide palliative care, 71% (n = 84) of the respondents felt sufficiently competent, and 12.7% (n = 15) felt that they are not sufficiently competent to provide palliative care. However, they must do it, and 16% (n = 19) answered "rarely", which suggests that their competence depends on the individual case. The participants were not, or were least involved in the inadequate provision of palliative care (M = 0.8; SD = 1.00). About 82% (n = 82) of the participants feel that the nursing home lacks the staff to provide quality care for the dying older person. Although nursing care is focused on the dying person, 73% (n = 73) of respondents felt that they did not have enough time to devote to the older person and their relatives, in the terminal phase.

Tab. 7.2: Frequency items for ethical issues during palliative care provision.

Frequency items (scale 0–5)	Never n(%)	Rarely n(%)	Often n(%)	Very often n(%)	M(SD)	EI
6. I have decided in the resident's best interest to prevent them from coming to harm or unnecessary risk.	0(0)	11(9.3)	20(16.9)	87(73.8)	3.09(0.99)	PI/IP
15. I have to follow the family's or care partner's wishes for the resident's care when I do not agree with them.	1(.8)	7(5.9)	32(27.1)	78(66.2)	2.77(0.85)	RI
5. I have to care for residents that only accept small amounts or refuse food and fluids near the end of life.	3(2.5)	15(12.7)	27(22.9)	73(61.9)	2.72(1.08)	RI
14. I witness distress from family or care partners.	7(5.9)	19(16.1)	19(16.1)	31(61.9)	2.60(1.20)	RI
20. I do not have enough time to provide the resident with the care she/he needs.	2(1.7)	17(14.4)	40(33.9)	59(50)	2.48(0.98)	OI
22. I find physician support lacking for resident care.	14(11.9)	20(16.9)	27(22.9)	57(48.3)	2.20(1.21)	OI
9. I have to initiate extensive life-saving actions when I think they only prolong death (e.g. PEG feeding, sub-cut fluids).	17(14.4)	22(18.6)	24(20.3)	55(46.7)	2.16(1.31)	PI/IP
24. I am involved in non-direct care activities, which reduce time spent with the residents.	14(11.9)	23(19.5)	29(24.6)	52(44)	2.14(1.21)	OI
1. I find it difficult to protect a resident's rights and dignity.	12(10.2)	28(23.7)	34(28.8)	44(37.3)	2.08(1.20)	PI/IP
7. I witness how poor staff communication diminishes the quality of care to residents.	11(9.3)	22(18.6)	44(37.3)	41(34.8)	2.05(1.06)	RI
4. I struggle to provide care to a resident due to their verbal or physical resistance.	13(11)	31(26.3)	32(27.1)	42(35.6)	2.03(1.23)	RI

Tab. 7.2 (continued)

Frequency items (scale 0–5)	Never n(%)	Rarely n(%)	Often n(%)	Very often n(%)	M(SD)	EI
3. I have to follow a request by a senior clinician not to discuss the resident's diagnosis with them when he/she asks for it.	27(22.9)	28(23.7)	21(17.8)	42(35.6)	1.85(1.45)	PI/IP
25. I feel the pain management is not satisfactory.	12(10.2)	35(29.7)	38(32.2)	33(27.9)	1.84(1.07)	OI
13. I feel powerless in decision-making during resident care.	17(14.4)	31(26.3)	34(28.8)	36(30.5)	1.82(1.15)	PI/IP
19. I cannot provide the care I want due to a lack of resources within the care home.	19(16.1)	38(32.2)	29(24.6)	32(27.1)	1.73(1.21)	OI
21. I cannot provide the quality of care I want due to conflicting care directions by external health and social care services.	17(14.4)	41(34.7)	31(26.3)	29(24.6)	1.72(1.19)	OI
8. I have observed professional incompetence due to insufficient staff training for providing nursing care.	19(16.1)	43(36.4)	27(22.9)	29(24.6)	1.62(1.13)	OI
2. At times, I have not been honest with a resident because I thought it was in their best interest.	19(16.1)	37(31.4)	38(32.2)	24(20.3)	1.61(1.07)	PI/IP
23. I have been involved in what felt like an unnecessary hospital admission.	24(20.3)	43(36.4)	24(20.4)	27(22.9)	1.57(1.25)	OI
12. I do not feel confident voicing my opinion regarding palliative care decisions.	25(21.2)	37(31.4)	32(27.1)	24(20.3)	1.54(1.18)	PI/IP
16. I am asked to provide care to the resident according to a senior clinician, specialist palliative care nurse, or charge nurse against my personal or professional opinion.	32(27.1)	42(35.6)	24(20.3)	20(17)	1.32(1.14)	RI
10. I do not know what care to provide, when no advance care plan has been agreed upon.	28(23.7)	45(38.1)	32(27.2)	13(11)	1.27(0.98)	PI/IP

Tab. 7.2 (continued)

Frequency items (scale 0–5)	Never n(%)	Rarely n(%)	Often n(%)	Very often n(%)	M(SD)	EI
18. I witness staff avoiding residents at the end of life due to their fears about dying.	29(24.6)	45(38.1)	30(25.4)	14(11.9)	1.27(1.01)	PI/IP
11. I do not know what to do when a senior clinician has provided unclear resident care instructions.	34(28.8)	43(36.4)	28(23.8)	13(11)	1.20(1.05)	PI/IP
17. I must provide palliative care for residents I do not feel trained to care for.	51(43.2)	33(28)	19(16.1)	15(12.7)	1.05(1.20)	OI
26. I have witnessed end-of-life care, which I felt was not satisfactory.	59(50)	35(29.7)	14(11.8)	10(8.5)	0.81(1)	OI

EI, ethical issues; n, sample size; OI, organizational issues; PI/IP, professional issues/issues in practice; RI, relational issues; SD, standard deviation.

7.4 Discussion

This study aims to determine the type and frequency of ethical issues among the nurses during the delivery of palliative care in nursing homes. Caring for older people needing palliative care brings on an emotional and psychological burden on the career; ethical issues appear, and it is difficult to manage them during such care [10]. The results showed that the most common ethical issues appear from the decision-making on behalf of the older people, in the areas of nutrition and hydration, family distress, and staff facing lack of time and poor communication between them.

Similarly, on the scale of frequency of occurrence, lack of time and too many non-patient-related activities are rated high (item 24). The ethical issue of reducing time to perform care is supported by Juthberg and Eriksson [19], who also found out that lack of time is associated with consciousness and causes stress, as the reduced time allocation to older people leads to the inability to perform person-centred care [4]. Older people's care in a nursing home must be comprehensive and person-centred, aiming to support older people's physical, social, spiritual, and psychological needs [2].

Many participants felt that the nursing home where they were employed provides person-centred care for the dying older person, but does not have enough time for the dying person to give full attention to them and their family. Research

[20] has shown that health professionals emphasise the safety of older people and do not allow them to make independent decisions about their health and themselves [20]. Our research agrees with the emphasis on care ethics, where the most common and difficult issues are related to ethical issues in practice and relational issues, including family distress, harm prevention, and respecting the family's wishes. To offer quality and comprehensive care, it is important to involve older people and their family members, early in the decision-making process [20].

It is also important that healthcare professionals trust each other and share decision-making power. Such an approach contributes to greater trust, reduction of ethical issues, and greater autonomy of older people. Not involving relatives in the medical treatment of older people causes stress, distress, and lack of strength and often leads to unhealthy hope. However, this unhealthy hope contributes to forcing unnecessary treatments and invasive procedures on older people needing palliative care. In this study and also Enes and de Vries [21], Schaffer [22], and Gjerberga et al. [23] found that interaction with family members is a concern for the nursing care team. Communication difficulties have led to challenges in decision-making and ethical issues in relationships, such as involving the patient and family in decision-making about care choices [9].

Communication problems cause feelings of not being heard, anger, helplessness, and bad conscience in older people, which has a fatal effect on individual healthcare professionals [2]. Results of our research showed how the family members' lack of support and involvement in the palliative care of their loved ones could contribute to unrealistic expectations in palliative care. The patient and family must be at the centre of the palliative care treatment, which can reduce unnecessary ethical issues.

Lopez [24] found that nurses feel they are between the physician and the family members in decision-making and are often doubtful about their role in providing care that will be acceptable to older people. In our study, we find out that older people, often, are not involved in the decision-making process of their own treatment when their ability to make decisions is questionable. Hence, the nurse plays an important role as an advocate of the wishes of the older people and, consequently, has an even greater role in making decisions in favour of the most vulnerable group of older people [2].

Among the organisational ethical issues, staff shortages and problems of inclusion of physicians in palliative care emerged as the biggest problems. Therefore, it is necessary to increase resources and improve the physicians' management of the care coordination in the palliative care of older people in nursing homes. Several problems involving the doctor have been reported in the literature.

Gágyor et al. [25] found that care coordination is limited even in homes with only one physician visit per week, and Enes and de Vries [21] found that the biggest ethical issue in nursing homes is the physician's lack of knowledge about symptom management. In contrast, Gágyor et al. [25] found that where there were more employed physicians, advanced guidelines were more often discussed at admission, and medical records were audited. Based on this, the older people made decisions in their treatment, and each healthcare professional was aware of their role and responsibility.

The health care team is crucial in ensuring the comfort of the dying person, as evidenced by the fact that very few nurses feel uncomfortable in performing nursing care, and there is little fear of death among them. They are trying to provide good care, even though they feel they do not have enough staff to provide effective nursing care. Although there are occasional shortages of resources within the institution, the dying person's care is adequately taken care. There is a definite shortage of staff in nursing homes, which is explained by the survey data of our research. As a result, nursing staff are more physically and mentally exhausted. Although care in care homes is centred on the dying older person, there is lack of time to devote fully to the dying older people and their relatives. Finally, poor staff communication and observation of professional incompetence reflect on staffing deficiencies, including a lack of knowledge, education and training on the extent of responsibility previously identified in the ethical literature in nursing homes [9, 25]. They may contribute to a reduction in the quality of care.

7.4.1 Limitations

Limitations of this research have been acknowledged. There may have been a non-response bias at the level of nursing homes, as those facing many ethical issues may not want to participate. Data was collected using a questionnaire, which means that there is a possibility that they gave socially desirable answers. Also, a relatively small sample was included in this study. All limitations need to be considered when interpreting the results.

7.5 Conclusion

The key ethical issues during the provision of palliative care in a nursing home include the autonomy of older people, family distress, lack of communication, lack of time, and staff incompetence. These findings have implications on nursing care practice in nursing homes, including how care is organized and the ability of nursing staff to care of older people needing palliative care. Many ethical issues can be solved by training staff to consider patient and family values, when making decisions consistent with global policy recommendations. Future research should explore these findings in more detail and use them to develop interventions that address these fundamental ethical issues. Nursing care homes should recognize and be attentive in order to identify ethical issues and educate their staff on how to resolve them.

References

[1] Benziger CP, Roth GA, Moran AE. The global burden of disease study and the preventable burden of NCD. Glob Heart, 2016, 11(4), 393–397.

[2] Preshaw DH, Brazil K, McLaughlin D, Frolic A. Ethical issues experienced by healthcare workers in nursing homes: Literature review. Nurs Ethics, 2016, 23(5), 490–506.

[3] Reitinger E, Froggatt K, Brazil K, Heimerl K, Hockley J, Kunz R, et al. Palliative care in long-term care settings for older people: Findings from an EAPC taskforce. Eur J Palliat Care, 2013, 20(5), 251–253.

[4] Kmetec S, Fekonja Z, Kolarič J, Reljić NM, McCormack B, Sigurðardóttir ÁK, et al. Components for providing person-centred palliative healthcare: An umbrella review. Int J Nurs Stud, 2022, 125, 104111.

[5] Reitinger E, Froggatt K, Brazil K, Heimerl K, Hockley J, Kunz R, et al. Palliative care in long-term care settings for older people: Findings from an EAPC taskforce. Eur J Palliat Care, 2013, 20, Epub.

[6] Lipman AG. Health literacy and palliative care: Workshop summary. J Pain Palliat Care Pharmacother, 2016, 30(3), 237–239.

[7] Kmetec S, Štiglic G, Lorber M, Mikkonen I, McCormack B, Pajnkihar M, et al. Nurses' perceptions of early person-centred palliative care: A cross-sectional descriptive study. Scand J Caring Sci, 2020, 34(1), 157–166.

[8] Leombruni P, Miniotti M, Bovero A, Castelli L, Torta R. Attitudes toward caring for dying patients: An overview among Italian nursing students and preliminary psychometrics of the FATCOD-B scale. J Nurs Educ Pract, 2013, 4, 188–196.

[9] Muldrew DHL, Kaasalainen S, McLaughlin D, Brazil K. Ethical issues in nursing home palliative care: A cross-national survey. BMJ Support Palliat Care, 2020, 10(3), e29.

[10] Preshaw DH, McLaughlin D, Brazil K. Ethical issues in palliative care for nursing homes: Development and testing of a survey instrument. J Clin Nurs, 2018, 27(3–4), e678–e87.

[11] Abudari G, Zahreddine H, Hazeim H, Assi MA, Emara S. Knowledge of and attitudes towards palliative care among multinational nurses in Saudi Arabia. Int J Palliat Nurs, 2014, 20(9), 435–441.

[12] Leclerc BS, Lessard S, Bechennec C, Le Gal E, Benoit S, Bellerose L. Attitudes toward death, dying, end-of-life palliative care, and interdisciplinary practice in long term care workers. J Am Med Dir Assoc, 2014, 15(3), 207–213.

[13] Simon ST, Ramsenthaler C, Bausewein C, Krischke N, Geiss G. Core attitudes of professionals in palliative care: A qualitative study. Int J Palliat Nurs, 2009, 15(8), 405–411.

[14] Lillemoen L, Pedersen R. Ethical challenges and how to develop ethics support in primary health care. Nurs Ethics, 2013, 20(1), 96–108.

[15] Polit D, Beck C. Nursing research: Generating and assessing evidence for nursing practice. 11th ed. Philadelphia, Wolters Kluwer, 2021.

[16] von Elm E, Altman DG, Egger M, Pocock SJ, Gøtzsche PC, Vandenbroucke JP. The strengthening the reporting of observational studies in epidemiology (STROBE) statement: Guidelines for reporting observational studies. PLoS Med, 2007, 4(10), e296.

[17] World Medical Association. Declaration of Helsinki. Ethical principles for medical research involving human subjects. Jahrbuch Für Wissenschaft Und Ethik, 2009, 14(1), 233–238.

[18] Council of Europe. Convention for the protection of human rights and dignity of the human beings with regard to the application of biology and medicine (European tratyseries-no. 164). Oviedo, Council of Europe.

[19] Juthberg C, Eriksson S, Norberg A, Sundin K. Perceptions of conscience, stress of conscience and burnout among nursing staff in residential elder care. J Adv Nurs, 2010, 66(8), 1708–1718.

[20] Cho HL, Grady C, Tarzian A, Povar G, Mangal J, Danis M. Patient and family descriptions of ethical concerns. Am J Bioeth, 2020, 20(6), 52–64.

[21] Enes SP, de Vries K. A survey of ethical issues experienced by nurses caring for terminally ill elderly people. Nurs Ethics, 2004, 11(2), 150–164.

[22] Schaffer MA. Ethical problems in end-of-life decisions for elderly Norwegians. Nurs Ethics, 2007, 14(2), 242–257.

[23] Gjerberg E, Førde R, Bjørndal A. Staff and family relationships in end-of-life nursing home care. Nurs Ethics, 2011, 18(1), 42–53.

[24] Lopez RP. Decision-making for acutely ill nursing home residents: Nurses in the middle. J Adv Nurs, 2009, 65(5), 1001–1009.

[25] Gágyor I, Heßling A, Heim S, Frewer A, Nauck F, Himmel W. Ethical challenges in primary care: A focus group study with general practitioners, nurses and informal caregivers. Fam Pract, 2019, 36(2), 225–230.

Barbara Kegl, Zvonka Fekonja, Sergej Kmetec,
Brendan McCormack, Nataša Mlinar Reljić

8 Elements of person-centred care of older people in primary healthcare: a systematic literature review with thematic analysis

Abstract

Background: Higher life expectancy in the ageing population and, consequently, an increase in the older population bring additional challenges for healthcare providers, especially in primary healthcare. The person-centred care of older people is defined as an approach that puts older people at the centre of care and recognizes the importance of their needs. The chapter aims to identify the key elements of person-centred care for older people, in primary healthcare.

Methods: A systematic review of relevant literature was carried out. Literature searches were conducted in international databases, with keywords and their synonyms with Boolean operators. The search was limited to articles published until December 2021.

Results: The literature review identified two main themes: (1) personal and communication determinants like the interaction of all participants, the experience of illness and the needs of the older people, the attitude of the primary healthcare team, the wishes of the older people; and (2) managerial characteristics that include qualification, leadership, organization, and operationalization.

Conclusion: The person-centred care of older people should be caring, compassionate, empathetic, confident, supportive, autonomous, and respectful. All these identified elements need to be heard and respected by all primary healthcare teams. It is important to recognize the needs of older people and, at the same time, have a positive experience with professional healthcare. The person-centred care of older people should focus on the patient's needs, family, and the wider local community.

Keywords: older people, primary healthcare team, health personnel, delivery of healthcare

8.1 Introduction

The world population is becoming increasingly older, life expectancy is rising [1], and the ageing population is the dominant demographic phenomenon of the 21st century [2]. The World Health Organization (WHO) states that by 2050, 80% of older people will live in low- and middle-income countries. Similar projections can also be seen in Slovenia, as the proportion of working for an active population in 2050 will account for only 50.5% of the total population. Higher life expectancy for the ageing population and the resulting increase in the older population brings additional challenges for all Western countries, due to increasing demand for efficient healthcare systems, especially in providing healthcare for an ageing population [3].

All countries face the significant challenges brought about by ageing and try to ensure that health and social systems are prepared for the greatest possible demographic change [4]. It is known that older people are frequent users of the healthcare system, especially in primary healthcare. Older people with chronic conditions receive person-centred primary healthcare from transdisciplinary healthcare teams, where care is often disorganized and confusing [5]. Primary healthcare teams are, often, the first healthcare professionals the older people consult or visit for their health problems [6].

Primary healthcare teams often face the increasing complexity of health conditions and the multimorbidity of older people [1]. Considering a multimorbidity of older people requires moving from disease-centred to person-centred healthcare. According to various authors, implementing person-centred healthcare means moving from the traditional biomedical model approach to an approach that emphasizes patient autonomy and participation in the treatment process [7]. The number of older people living at home will increase dramatically due to demographic changes [8]. With age, chronic non-communicable disease increases. At the same time, people experience a decline in physical and mental abilities, leading to losing functional abilities that is challenging for the primary care team [9]. Person-centred healthcare outlines a standard of care that puts older people at the centre of events and recognizes the importance of their knowledge and experience [10]. Older people are included as partners in their healthcare planning and disease control, with decisions that take into account their individual needs, values, and preferences [11]. Research shows that person-centred healthcare for older people improves their quality of life, provides better quality healthcare [12], and is linked to greater satisfaction of both users and providers of such care [13].

The person-centred healthcare approach for older people is highly recommended by World Health Organization [4] and McCormack [7] as a means to improve the standards of healthcare [14]. The current use of person-centred primary healthcare in family medicine is effective, because patients better manage their health by changing their lifestyles [15]. However, its implementation in practice is limited, and it also relates to the characteristics of the patient and the primary healthcare team. A primary healthcare team comprises a team of healthcare professionals, who work closely together to provide care and support to older people living in the community [16]. Therefore, to implement such an approach, we want to identify important elements of person-centred healthcare for older people and provide guidelines for such an approach in primary healthcare.

8.2 Methods

A systematic review was conducted using the methods of analysis, synthesis, and compilation of the literature. This methodological approach allows analysis, synthesis of knowledge, and applicability of results to practice. The process of searching and data extraction of the paper was guided by the Preferred Reporting Items for Systematic Reviews (PRISMA) [17] recommendations and is presented in the flow diagram (Fig. 8.1).

8.2.1 Research question

For the systematic review, we developed a PIO question: Which person-centred healthcare elements (I) impact the effectiveness of caring (O) for older people (P) in primary healthcare?

8.2.2 Search strategy

Literature searching took place in December 2021 in the following databases: PubMed, CINAHL, MEDLINE, and ScienceDirect by using search terms in English: person-centred healthcare, elements, impact, caring, older people, primary healthcare, and their synonyms with Boolean operators (AND/OR). The obtained results from databases were imported into the program, EndNote 20, and examined according to the eligibility criteria (Tab. 8.1).

Tab. 8.1: The eligibility criteria for systematic review.

Databases	PubMed, CINAHL, MEDLINE, and ScienceDirect	
	Inclusion criteria	Exclusion criteria
Participants	– Older people (+65 years)	– A person younger than 65 years
Intervention/ treatment	– Person-centred healthcare	– Exclude person-centred healthcare
Outcome	– Effectiveness of person-centred healthcare for older people at primary healthcare	– Exclude the effectiveness of person-centred healthcare for older people in primary healthcare

Tab. 8.1 (continued)

Databases	PubMed, CINAHL, MEDLINE, and ScienceDirect	
	Inclusion criteria	**Exclusion criteria**
Types of research	– Research article (quantitative, qualitative, and mixed methods research)	– Systematic review articles or other types of reviews – Duplicates, commentaries, editorials, conferences, and research protocols – Reviews that do not relate to our PIO question
Search limits		
Timeframe	Until December 2021	
Language	English or Slovenian	

8.2.3 Methodology assessment

The "Joanna Briggs Institute (JBI) Critical Appraisal Checklist" (2019) was critically evaluated for methodological quality. To assess the quality of the papers, we used the JBI Critical Appraisal Checklist for (i) qualitative research [18]; (ii) analytical cross-sectional research [19]; and (iii) randomized controlled trials [20]. JBI quality assessment tools include methodological appraisal questions that help authors determine the methodological rigour of included studies. For each of the checklists used, the answers were scored: "Yes" got one point; "No", and "Unclear" got zero points. After the assessment, we calculated the sum and percentage of all points for each study. Based on the authors, Camp and Legge's [21] recommendation, we evaluated and divided the studies into four groups: low quality (60–69%); medium quality (70–79%); high quality (80–90%); and excellent quality (more than 90%).

8.2.4 Data extraction and synthesis

The data extraction was conducted based on predefined data extraction criteria (e.g., authors, year, country, andpurpose). The data synthesis was based on a thematic framework by Thomas and Harden [22]. The first author read the text line by line based on each paper's identified free codes. These free codes were then organized in a descriptive primary subtheme and analysed and compared with one another to develop a secondary theme in the MAXQDA Analytics Pro-program. Co-authors reviewed the thematic synthesis, and any disagreements were resolved through discussion and consensus.

8.3 Results

8.3.1 Selection of relevant papers

With the help of the search strategy and limits of the search, we found 4 PubMed records, 4 CINAHL records, 4 MEDLINE records, 60 ScienceDirect records, and 3,557 Wiley Online Library records. After that, we eliminated 779 duplicates. The next step was that two reviewers searched the titles and abstracts of the results independently, depending on the limitations. The next step was to read the full articles and include or exclude the paper, depending on the limitations. According to the appropriateness of the content, we eliminated 39 hits out of 52 fully available papers. We eliminated them because they did not include patients older than 65 years and did not relate to the searched topic. The final number of useful records was 13 papers (Fig. 8.1).

8.3.2 Characteristics of papers

We included 13 studies in a review of the literature related to the approach of the person-centred healthcare of older people in primary healthcare. Nine studies used a qualitative research approach and four, quantitative studies. In qualitative research, four studies used individual interviews, three used focus groups, and two used an observation method. Quantitative studies used questionnaires as a research tool, and two were randomized control trials. A detailed description of each study is shown in Tab. 8.2.

8.3.3 Critical assessment

Details of critical assessment are shown in tables. Five papers were evaluated as medium quality [25, 26, 28, 31, 32], six of them were graded as high quality [6, 11, 23, 27, 29, 30], and two were excellent quality [24, 33] (Tab. 8.3).

8.3.4 Results of data synthesis

To identify the key elements of person-centred primary healthcare for older people, each paper (n =13) was coded line by line, and free codes were established (n = 119). Free codes were then combined in the descriptive primary level subthemes (n = 19), and with their analysis and comparison, secondary level subthemes were developed (n = 7). All themes were synthesized and developed, from which we identified two main themes: (1) the primary healthcare process and (2) person-centred leadership elements (Fig. 8.2).

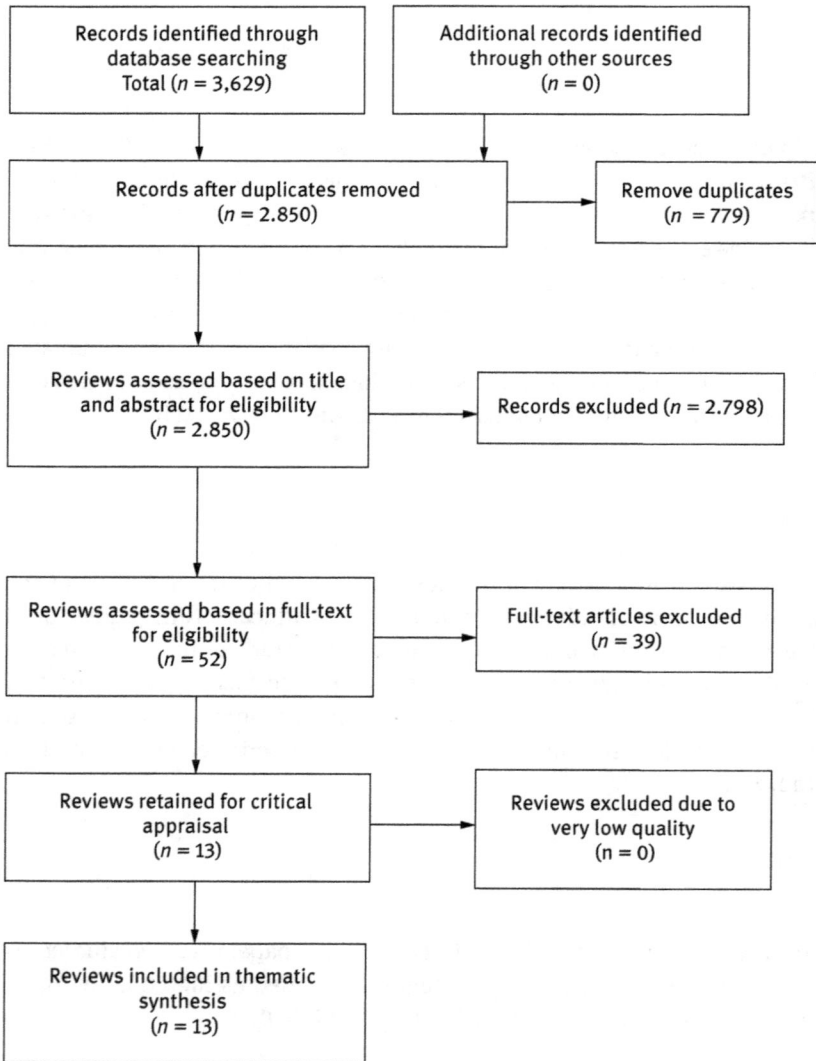

Fig. 8.1: The process of selecting the studies.

The primary healthcare process

Within the primary healthcare process, we have identified four secondary level sub-themes that relate to the person-centred healthcare of older people in primary healthcare: (1) interaction of all participants; (2) the experience of diseases and the needs of the older people; (3) primary healthcare team relationship; and (4) wishes of the older people.

Tab. 8.2: Characteristics of included papers.

Author, country	Research design	Aim of research	Sample size	Main findings related to detected symptoms
Sarkisian et al. [23], USA	Qualitative study; focus group	To compare the expectations of older people and physicians as regards their visits	$n = 49$ older people than 65 years and $n = 11$ physicians of primary healthcare	– The most commonly reported problematic areas about reasons for their visits are physical function, cognitive function, social function, pain, and sexual function – Older people expressed that they felt like numbers and not like people, nor were they involved in decision-making – The physician stared at the computer throughout the conversation and did not make eye contact
Shields et al. [24], USA	Quantitative study; randomized control study	To examine the interaction between the physician and the accompanied older people	$n = 13$ older people with an accompanying person and $n = 17$ without an accompanying person	– Physicians talked for a long time without a break with those who have had a companion because they thought such a visit was more complex and required more explanation – Physicians equally carefully followed the patient's health problems and talked to them about diagnosis and treatment, irrespective of whether they were patients with or without an escort – Escorting a family member or friend does not result in less attention by the physician and does not divert the physician's attention from the patient

Tab. 8.2 (continued)

Author, country	Research design	Aim of research	Sample size	Main findings related to detected symptoms
Bastiaens et al. [6], Belgium Slovenia Portugal UK and Northern Ireland	Qualitative study; interviews	To explore the views of people aged 70 and over on their involvement in primary healthcare in 11 European countries	$n = 406$ older people aged between 70 and 96	– Older people want to be involved in their care and be involved in decision-making. However, their definition of integration focuses on a loving relationship, a person-centred approach, receiving information, communication, and support – The study stresses the importance of good communication, including interest in the problem, clear information, and being reliable and supportive
Smith and Orrell [25], UK and Northern Ireland	Quantitative study; Cross-Sectional Study	Analyse the impact of a person-centred approach in the general practice clinic to identify unfulfilled needs in older people	$n = 67$ older people older than 65 years	– The person-centred approach was very much appreciated but is not associated with reduced unfulfilled needs – Many older peoples tolerate unfulfilled needs, and they are reluctant to acknowledge or mention that to their physician – The most frequent unfulfilled needs were: information (19%), vision/hearing/communication (16%), and physical health (16%)

Tab. 8.2 (continued)

Author, country	Research design	Aim of research	Sample size	Main findings related to detected symptoms
Bayliss et al. [26], USA	Qualitative study; Interviews	Explore the approach of healthcare for older people with multimorbidity	$n = 26$ older people aged between 65 and 84	– Older people try to find such care that includes: the need for convenient access/making an appointment at the physician (phone, internet, or in-person), clear communication including an individualized plan of health care, support by the healthcare team who could help support the needs of older people and continuity of relationship – it is important for them to be heard and understood – They also want healthcare workers who will listen to them and recognize their needs, identify them as unique and can fluctuate, and have a caring attitude towards them – Older people want more information on managing chronic conditions such as diabetes or the results of various laboratory tests
Berkelmans et al. [27], Netherlands	Qualitative study; interviews	Improve understanding of wishes and expectations of older people regarding non-health characteristics of primary healthcare	$n = 13$ older people aged between 65 and 91	– The older people greatly appreciate the following: continuous healthcare (physicians and nurses), medical expertise, free choice of physicians, trust, and an open attitude – Respondents indicate problems with the 24-h service – The respondents prefer to receive verbal information over information from brochures

Tab. 8.2 (continued)

Author, country	Research design	Aim of research	Sample size	Main findings related to detected symptoms
Wolff and Roter [28], USA	Qualitative study; observation	To explore whether the presence of a family member as a companion in a routine examination with the family physician helps or hinders the person-centred care of older people process	Older people older than 65 years and their family members (n = 390 – n = 80 older people accompanied and n = 310 older people unaccompanied)	– Older people with poor mental health, whom a family member accompanied, the patient gave less psycho-social information, physicians asked less and tried to establish an interpersonal relationship – – Both the patient and the physician had a more task-oriented biomedical discussion – Older people with poor mental health with an attendant were less likely to have received person-centred communication than the unaccompanied patients
Fried et al. [29], USA	Qualitative study; focus groups	Explore the views and experiences of clinical staff (physicians and nurses) with therapeutic decision-making in older people patients with multiple health problems	n = 40 healthcare professionals	– Participants were concerned about the ability to cope with a complex regime of treatment for older people – Participants indicated several obstacles to good clinical decisions, and these involve a lack of information on the results of treatment, the role of a specialist, the expectations of patients and families, the lack of time, and reimbursement of expenses

Tab. 8.2 (continued)

Author, country	Research design	Aim of research	Sample size	Main findings related to detected symptoms
van de Pol et al. [30], Netherlands	Qualitative study; focus groups	To explore the main areas for improving older people's healthcare from healthcare professionals and older people in primary healthcare	$n = 53$ older people older than 80 years; $n = 20$ physicians and $n = 21$ nurses	– Participants stressed the importance to clarify different views regarding good health-care among patients and healthcare professionals – Effective interventions for older people require a mutual understanding of the expectations and goals of all involved in primary healthcare – Several requirements were identified, particularly access to information and medical treatment planning, training of health professionals about complex healthcare and multimorbidity, autonomy, setting targets, and common concerns
Bogner et al. [31], USA	Quantitative study; cross-sectional study	Explore the level of older people's satisfaction and perceived quality of health services related to the level of activities of daily living	$n = 42.584$ older people aged more than 65 years	– Respondents were satisfied with the physician's quality of work within the meaning of perceived technical and interpersonal skills and delivering information – More than 80% of older people were very satisfied or satisfied. More than 90% reported that they were very satisfied or satisfied with the quality of care and the technical skills of primary care physicians – It is necessary to use such strategies, including the perception of patients and evaluation of quality assurance

Tab. 8.2 (continued)

Author, country	Research design	Aim of research	Sample size	Main findings related to detected symptoms
Coulourides Kogan et al. [11], USA	Qualitative study; interviews	Obtain the views and experience of implementing such care by the heads of health services at the primary healthcare	The study invited 18 organizations, of which 9 took part in the survey	– There were three identified topics regarding implementing person-centred care of older people (PCC): operationalization (including environmental, attributes of supply and measurement), feasibility, challenges, and language – Older people consider PCC to be quality care and have expressed a strong preference for a PCC that focuses on their needs, puts their preferences first, and addresses the problems that older people identify
Wolff et al. [32], USA	Qualitative study; observation	Explore the communication behaviour of family companions while older people visit their physician	Visits of the older people at the general practice accompanied by a family companion ($n = 30$ visits)	– Family attendants largely facilitated the flow of information between physician and patient – The attendants were more verbally active in visits of the older people who have managed their health with the help of others than in other visits to the older people who were partially dependent or independent in managing their health – Attendants evaluated that they felt more helpful with those older people who want the active involvement of the family in the decision-making process about their health

Tab. 8.2 (continued)

Author, country	Research design	Aim of research	Sample size	Main findings related to detected symptoms
Uittenbroek et al. [33], Netherlands	Quantitative study; randomized control study	Examine the effectiveness of the Embrace program and integrated primary healthcare services for older people	A total of 1,456 older people who have a family physician participated, in 15 clinics	− After 12 months, the Embrace program showed that PCC does not affect the cost increase. − They note that Embrace and the standard treatment increase the cost of treatment in older people; therefore, only one must be used to improve the risk profile − Older people must be provided with such treatment to deal with their complex medical needs

Tab. 8.3: A critical assessment of included papers.

JBI CA checklist CS	1	2	3	4	5	6	7	8	QS
Including papers (n = 2)									
Bogner [31]	Y	Y	Y	Y	U	U	Y	Y	6/8
Smith and Orrell [25]	Y	Y	Y	Y	U	N	Y	Y	6/8

CS, cross-sectional studies; CA, critical appraisal; Y, yes; N, no; U, unclear; NA, not applicable; QS, quality score.
1. Were the criteria for inclusion in the sample clearly defined?
2. Were the study subjects and the setting described in detail?
3. Was the exposure measured validly and reliably?
4. Were objective, standard criteria used for measurement of the condition?
5. Were confounding factors identified?
6. Were strategies to deal with confounding factors stated?
7. Were the outcomes measured validly and reliably?
8. Was appropriate statistical analysis used?

JBI CA checklist QR	1	2	3	4	5	6	7	8	9	10	QS
Including papers (n = 9)											
Sarkisian et al. [23]	Y	Y	Y	Y	Y	N	U	Y	Y	Y	8/10
Bastiaens et al. [6]	Y	Y	Y	Y	Y	U	Y	Y	Y	Y	9/10
Bayliss et al. [26]	N	Y	Y	Y	Y	U	N	Y	Y	Y	7/10

Tab. 8.3 (continued)

JBI CA checklist QR	1	2	3	4	5	6	7	8	9	10	QS
Including papers (n = 9)											
Berkelmans et al. [27]	Y	Y	Y	Y	Y	N	U	Y	Y	Y	8/10
Wolff and Roter [28]	U	Y	Y	Y	Y	U	N	Y	Y	Y	7/10
Fried et al. [29]	Y	Y	Y	Y	Y	N	N	Y	Y	Y	8/10
Van de Pol et al. [30]	Y	Y	Y	Y	Y	N	Y	Y	Y	Y	9/10
Coulourides Kogan et al. [11]	U	Y	Y	Y	Y	U	Y	Y	Y	Y	8/10
Wolff et al. [32]	Y	Y	Y	Y	Y	N	N	Y	N	Y	7/10

QR, qualitative research; CA, critical appraisal; Y, yes; N, no; U, unclear; NA, not applicable.
1. Is there congruity between the stated philosophical perspective and the research methodology?
2. Is there congruity between the research methodology and the research question or objectives?
3. Is there congruity between the research methodology and the methods used to collect data?
4. Is there congruity between the research methodology and the representation and analysis of data?
5. Is there congruity between the research methodology and the interpretation of results?
6. Is there a statement locating the researcher culturally or theoretically?
7. Is the researcher's influence on the research, and vice versa, addressed?
8. Are participants, and their voices, adequately represented?
9. Is the research ethical according to current criteria o, for recent studies, and is there evidence of ethical approval by an appropriate body?
10. Do the conclusions drawn in the research report flow from the data's analysis or interpretation?

JBI CA checklist RCT	1	2	3	4	5	6	7	8	9	10	11	12	13	QS
Including papers (n = 2)														
Shields et al. [24]	Y	Y	Y	Y	Y	Y	Y	Y	Y	Y	Y	Y	Y	13/13
Uittenbroek et al. [33]	Y	Y	Y	Y	Y	Y	Y	Y	Y	Y	Y	Y	Y	13/13

RCT, randomized control trial; CA, critical appraisal; Y, yes; N, no; U, unclear; NA, not applicable.
1. Was true randomization used to assign participants to treatment groups?
2. Was allocation to treatment groups concealed?
3. Were treatment groups similar at the baseline?
4. Were participants blind to treatment assignment?
5. Were those delivering treatment blind to treatment assignment?
6. Were outcomes assessors blind to treatment assignment?
7. Were treatment groups treated identically other than the intervention of interest?
8. Was follow up complete and if not, were differences between groups in terms of their follow-up adequately described and analysed?
9. Were participants analysed in the groups to which they were randomized?
10. Were outcomes measured in the same way for treatment groups?
11. Were outcomes measured in a reliable way?
12. Was appropriate statistical analysis used?
13. Was the trial design appropriate, and were any deviations from the standard RCT design (individual randomization, parallel groups) accounted for in the conduct and analysis of the trial?

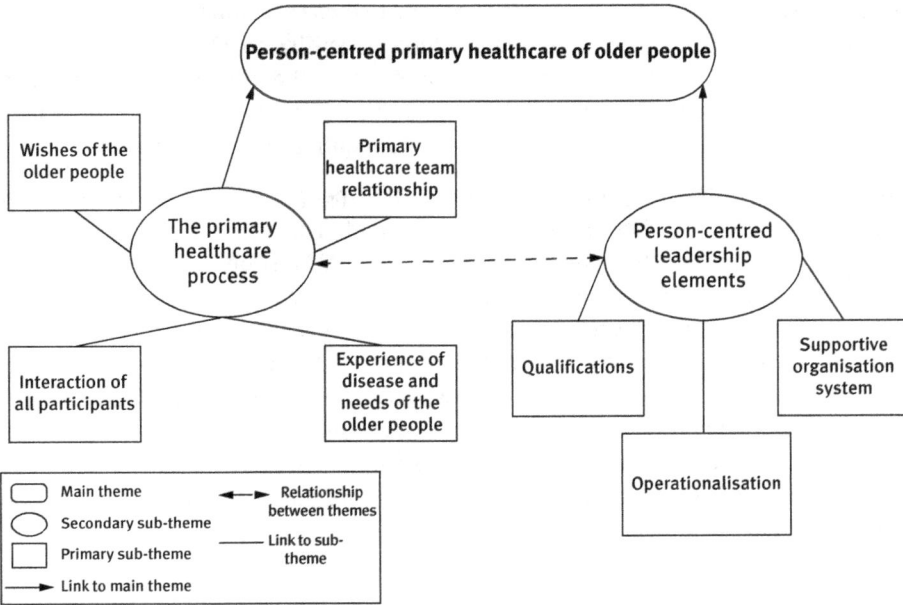

Fig. 8.2: The results from data synthesis with main theme and subthemes.

Interaction of all participants: Interaction of all participants includes three elements: information, communication, and interpersonal relations. Older people appreciate good [6] and clear communication [26], which should be reflected in showing interest in their health problems and giving information to them in an appropriate manner [6]. Furthermore, older people most often wish to receive clear information [6, 26, 30] from healthcare professionals, but the information must be given in person by healthcare professionals [27] and compassionately [31].

Experience of disease and needs of the older people: The experience of disease and the needs of older people are composed of two elements: emotional and physical needs. The primary healthcare team must identify and prioritize the issues and problems of older people [11, 30, 33]. Sarkisian et al. [23] describe the most frequent problem areas such as physical, cognitive, social, and sexual function, and pain. Furthermore, additional areas related to mental health: anxiety, emotional well-being, happiness, sleep, and life/death are mentioned.

Primary healthcare team relationship: The primary healthcare team relationship consists of two elements: the process of the visit and the outcome of the visit. Older people often visit their physician with a companion, who is their family member or friend [28, 32]. Bastiaens et al. [6] found that an accompanied visit in the form of a care partner does not result in decreased attention by the physician, or the attention is not diverted away from the older people. On the other hand, Wolff and Roter [28] conclude that the physician asks fewer questions to those accompanying older people and tries to establish interpersonal relationships. According to Shields et al. [24], the companions effectively direct the conversation between the primary healthcare team and the older people by opening new issues; for this reason, according to the primary healthcare team, such a visit is more complex and requires more explanation.

Wishes of the older people: Wishes of the older people include three elements: personal, primary healthcare team, and treatment. The views and wishes of the older people regarding their treatment were different. Most often, they want a caring [6, 30] and an open attitude [27], which is believed to be characterized by trust, support, interest, respect, understanding, and listening [6, 24, 26, 30]. The physician must answer their questions, listen to them, have time for them, put their wishes first, involve them in the care, and recognize their needs as unique [6, 26, 30]. Their treatment should be based on mutual understanding and common determination of goals [30], the recognition of their needs [26], and maintaining their autonomy and independence [30]. They also want to spend more time with their chosen physician [30], whom they can choose by themselves [27].

Person-centred leadership elements

Within the person-centred leadership elements, three secondary-level subthemes have been identified: (1) qualifications; (2) supportive organization system; and (3) operationalization.

Qualifications: Qualification is composed of two elements: expertise and skill. Successful performance and quality of care of older people require expertise of the primary healthcare team [24, 25]. The primary healthcare team must have the skills to deal with the complex health problems of older people and treatment regimes [29]; that is why, it is important to train them [30]. The older people expressed most satisfaction with their technical and interpersonal skills, because they feel that their problems are understood and considered by the primary healthcare team [31].

Supportive organization system: The supportive organization system comprises quality, accessibility, and obstacles. Experience of the older people with their healthcare is reflected in satisfaction and dissatisfaction. Older people were satisfied with the quality of provided care but dissatisfied with care coordination, access, and visit coordination [31]. Most obstacles to implementing person-centred primary healthcare for older people have been noted in finance, structure and overburdening of staff, the organization, and the rigidity of staff [25]. Older people have expressed their desire for convenient access or appointment with a physician by telephone, Internet, or in person [24, 27, 30]. They highly appreciate primary healthcare team visits at home [24] and the support of the healthcare coordinator [11, 26].

Operationalization: The operationalization consists of two elements: form and views. Primary healthcare teams and the older people perceived person-centred healthcare of older people differently. They emphasized the importance of clarifying different views regarding good healthcare between older people and the primary healthcare team [30]. According to Coulorides Kogan et al. [11], the most frequently reported features of patient-centred healthcare are teamwork care, multidisciplinary care, electronic documentation, and care coordination. Furthermore, Coulorides Kogan et al. [11] strongly prefer this approach, because it follows the patient's health problems [24]. In practice, this means implementing continuous care [27], where the interpersonal relationship is independent of the wishes and capabilities of older people being part of the decision-making process [6].

8.4 Discussion

A literature review provided broader insight into elements of person-centred primary healthcare for older people. We identify two key elements of providing person-centred primary healthcare for older people: The primary healthcare process and person-centred leadership elements (see Fig. 8.2). The person-centred care of older people is commonly reported in healthcare literature [34, 35]. It is defined as the preferred approach to the healthcare of older people. However, there is little consensus on its definition, measurement, factors, or association with better health outcomes for individuals [34]. Person-centred care is defined as delivering respectful care and responding to older people's needs and values [36].

Furthermore, it adjusts the care according to the needs of older people [7], understanding the older people as unique human beings and seeing the person as a whole [37]. A literature analysis showed that older people wish for autonomy [30] and involvement in decision-making [6]. At the same time, they want continuity of care and focus on themselves, which allows them to follow up on their health problems and wishes [6, 24, 29].

In the reviewed literature, we have identified specific elements of the person-centred primary healthcare of older people and skills that affect the entire process of healthcare: convenient access to providers of healthcare services (e.g. phone, internet, or in-person), clear communication (e.g., preferably in writing), individualized advance care plan, older people's chosen primary physician who knows them, and respect of primary healthcare team.

Primary healthcare teams face many older people with multimorbidity and complex healthcare needs [38, 39]. One of the many challenges at the primary healthcare level is providing structured and well-coordinated care [38–40]. Bayliss et al. [26] note that older people want the support of primary healthcare teams, which help them prioritize their health problems and provide continuity of care. Primary healthcare teams should take a holistic approach to the following-up of older people, focusing on the following elements: appropriate communication (e.g., accessibility and empathy), cooperation and partnership, and the provision of clear information [25, 26, 30].

Person-centred primary healthcare of older people should be carried out in such a way that it is caring, compassionate, and empathetic. It puts older people in the spotlight, is unique to the individual's needs, and considers the older people as part of their care. Older people wish for a caring attitude, confidence, support, autonomy, independence, and respect, and they want to be heard and understood. All these elements need to be noted and respected by all primary healthcare teams, so that they can carry out diligent and person-centred primary healthcare for older people.

8.4.1 Strengths and limitations

Our strength lies in that we have followed the recommendation for conducting a literature review by Hannes [41]. Furthermore, we have conducted systematic and detailed search in databases, data extraction, quality assessment, and thematic analysis of the included studies. All steps of our literature review are represented in the tables and figures. However, a limitation of some studies can be the sample size and process of sampling for the research. Although we had access to many papers, some important articles were probably excluded, based on our inclusion criteria. The review included only papers with the specific search terms used. The weakness is that we may not have reviewed all the relevant literature, because we could have used other additional search synonyms. Nevertheless, we believe these identified records are large enough to prove and support our results.

8.4.2 Implications for research and practice

Further research is needed to determine the influence of person-centred primary healthcare and the decision of older people to obtain an emergency department rather than their primary healthcare team. Increasing numbers of older people patients call for well-organized primary healthcare at the local and national level, considering the older people's position, encouraging empowerment, and placing it at the centre of healthcare. Analysis of the literature has helped us easily identify the needs of older people at the primary healthcare level: the interaction of all stakeholders, the experience of disease and needs, attitude of a primary healthcare team, wishes of older people, and person-centred leadership. These identified elements of person-centred primary healthcare for older people have a significant impact on developing a modern healthcare strategy, meeting the older people's needs, and positively impacting their experience. Person-centred primary healthcare for older people should reflect interprofessional and evidence-based healthcare, which will be focused on older people, their family members, and the wider local community.

References

[1]   Day H, Eckstrom E, Lee S, Wald H, Counsell S, Rich E. Optimizing health for complex adults in primary care: current challenges and a way forward. J Gen Intern Med, 2014, 29(6), 911–914.

[2]   Bloom DE, Luca DL. Chapter 1 – the global demography of aging: Facts, explanations, future. In: Piggott J, Woodland A, eds. Handbook of the economics of population aging. 1. North-Holland, Amsterdam 2016, 3–56.

[3]   Kavaš D, Koman K, Kump N, Majcen B, Sambt J, Stropnik N. Spodbujanje podaljšanega zaposlovanja in odloženega upokojevanja: Analiza obstoječih politik in predlog ukrepov. Ljubljana, Inštitut za ekonomska raziskovanja, 2016.

[4]   World Health Organization. Towards people-centred health systems: An innovative approach for better health outcomes. Copenhagen, World Health Organization, 2013.

[5]   Elliot AJ, Heffner KL, Mooney CJ, Moynihan JA, Chapman BP. Social relationships and inflammatory markers in the MIDUS cohort: The role of age and gender differences. J Aging Health, 2017, 30(6), 904–923.

[6]   Bastiaens H, Van Royen P, Pavlic DR, Raposo V, Baker R. Older people's preferences for involvement in their own care: A qualitative study in primary healthcare in 11 European countries. Patient Educ Couns, 2007, 68(1), 33–42.

[7]   McCormack B, McCance T, Bulley C, Brown D, McMillan A, Martin S. Fundamentals of person-centred healthcare practice. Hoboken, Wiley-Blackwell, 2021.

[8]   Van Dijk HM, Cramm JM, Van Exel JOB, Nieboer AP. The ideal neighbourhood for ageing in place as perceived by frail and non-frail community-dwelling older people. Ageing Soc, 2015, 35(8), 1771–1795.

[9]   Asogwa OA, Boateng D, Marzà-Florensa A, Peters S, Levitt N, van Olmen J, et al. Multimorbidity of non-communicable diseases in low-income and middle-income countries: A systematic review and meta-analysis. BMJ Open, 2022, 12(1), e049133.

[10] Thiengtham S, D'Avolio D, Leethong-in M. Family involvement in transitional care from hospital to home and its impact on older patients, families, and healthcare providers: A mixed methods systematic review protocol. JBI Evidence Synth, 2022, 20(2), 606–612.

[11] Coulourides Kogan A, Wilber K, Mosqueda L. Moving toward implementation of person-centred care for older adults in community-based medical and social service settings: "You only get things done when working in concert with clients". J Am Geriatr Soc, 2016, 64(1), e8–e14.

[12] Kmetec S, Fekonja Z, Kolarič JČ, Reljić NM, McCormack B, Sigurðardóttir ÁK, et al. Components for providing person-centred palliative healthcare: An umbrella review. Int J Nurs Stud, 2022, 125, 104111.

[13] Ekman I, Wolf A, Olsson LE, Taft C, Dudas K, Schaufelberger M, et al. Effects of person-centred care in patients with chronic heart failure: The PCC-HF study. Eur Heart J, 2012, 33(9), 1112–1119.

[14] Laird EA, McCance T, McCormack B, Gribben B. Patients' experiences of in-hospital care when nursing staff were engaged in a practice development programme to promote person-centredness: A narrative analysis study. Int J Nurs Stud, 2015, 52(9), 1454–1462.

[15] Delaney LJ. Patient-centred care as an approach to improving healthcare in Australia. Collegian, 2018, 25(1), 119–123.

[16] Galvez-Hernandez P, González-de Paz L, Muntaner C. Primary care-based interventions addressing social isolation and loneliness in older people: A scoping review. BMJ Open, 2022, 12(2), e057729.

[17] Moher D, Altman DG, Liberati A, Tetzlaff J. PRISMA statement. Epidemiology, 2011, 22(1), 128.

[18] Lockwood C, Munn Z, Porritt K. Qualitative research synthesis: Methodological guidance for systematic reviewers utilising meta-aggregation. JBI Evidence Implementation, 2015, 13(3), 179–187.

[19] Moola S, Munn Z, Tufanaru C, Aromataris E, Sears K, Sfetcu R, et al. Chapter 7: Systematic reviews of etiology and risk. In: Joanna Briggs institute reviewer's manual [Internet]. Adelaide, The Joanna Briggs Institute, 2017, Available from: https://synthesismanual.jbi.global.

[20] Tufanaru C, Munn Z, Aromataris E, Campbell J, Hopp L. Chapter 3: Systematic reviews of effectiveness. In: Joanna Briggs institute reviewer's manual [Internet]. Adelaide, Joanna Briggs Institute, 2017, Available from: https://synthesismanual.jbi.global/.

[21] Camp S, Legge T. Simulation as a tool for clinical remediation: An integrative review. Clin Simul Nurs, 2018, 16, 48–61.

[22] Thomas J, Harden A. Methods for the thematic synthesis of qualitative research in systematic reviews. BMC Med Res Methodol, 2008, 8(1), 1–10.

[23] Sarkisian CA, Hays RD, Berry SH, Mangione CM. Expectations regarding aging among older adults and physicians who care for older adults. Med Care, 2001, 39(9), 1025–1036.

[24] Shields CG, Epstein RM, Fiscella K, Franks P, McCann R, McCormick K, et al. Influence of accompanied encounters on patient-centeredness with older patients. J Am Board Fam Pract, 2005, 18(5), 344–354.

[25] Smith F, Orrell M. Does the patient-centred approach help identify the needs of older people attending primary care? Age Ageing, 2007, 36(6), 628–631.

[26] Bayliss EA, Edwards AE, Steiner JF, Main DS. Processes of care desired by elderly patients with multimorbidities. Fam Pract, 2008, 25(4), 287–293.

[27] Berkelmans PG, Berendsen AJ, Verhaak PFM, van der Meer K. Characteristics of general practice care: What do senior citizens value? A qualitative study. BMC Geriatr, 2010, 10(1), 80.

[28] Wolff JL, Roter DL. Older adults' mental health function and patient-centred care: Does the presence of a family companion help or hinder communication? J Gen Intern Med, 2012, 27(6), 661–668.

[29] Fried TR, Tinetti ME, Iannone L. Primary care clinicians' experiences with treatment decision making for older persons with multiple conditions. Arch Intern Med, 2011, 171(1), 75–80.

[30] van de Pol MH, Fluit CR, Lagro J, Niessen D, Rikkert MG, Lagro-Janssen AL. Quality care provision for older people: An interview study with patients and primary healthcare professionals. Br J Gen Pract, 2015, 65(637), e500–e507.

[31] Bogner HR, de Vries Mcclintock HF, Hennessy S, Kurichi JE, Streim JE, Xie D, et al. Patient satisfaction and perceived quality of care among older adults according to activity limitation stages. Arch Phys Med Rehabil, 2015, 96(10), 1810–1819.

[32] Wolff JL, Guan Y, Boyd CM, Vick J, Amjad H, Roth DL, et al. Examining the context and helpfulness of family companion contributions to older adults' primary care visits. Patient Educ Couns, 2017, 100(3), 487–494.

[33] Uittenbroek RJ, van Asselt ADI, Spoorenberg SLW, Kremer HPH, Wynia K, Reijneveld SA. Integrated and person-centred care for community-living older adults: A cost-effectiveness study. Health Serv Res, 2018, 53(5), 3471–3494.

[34] Bertakis KD, Azari R. Patient-centred care is associated with decreased healthcare utilisation. J Am Board Fam Med, 2011, 24(3), 229–239.

[35] Edvardsson D, Nay R. Acute care and older people: Challenges and ways forward. Aust J Adv Nurs, 2009, 27, 63–69.

[36] Baker A. Institute of Medicine (US) Committee on Quality of Health Care in America. Crossing the Quality Chasm: A New Health System for the 21st Century. Washington: National Academies Press; 2001

[37] Martínez T, Postigo Á, Cuesta M, Muñiz J. Person-centred care for older people: Convergence and assessment of users' relatives' and staff's perspectives. J Adv Nurs, 2021, 77(6), 2916–2927.

[38] Bower P, Macdonald W, Harkness E, Gask L, Kendrick T, Valderas JM, et al. Multimorbidity, service organization and clinical decision making in primary care: A qualitative study. Fam Pract, 2011, 28(5), 579–587.

[39] Glynn LG, Valderas JM, Healy P, Burke E, Newell J, Gillespie P, et al. The prevalence of multimorbidity in primary care and its effect on healthcare utilisation and cost. Fam Pract, 2011, 28(5), 516–523.

[40] Mercer SW, Smith SM, Wyke S, O'Dowd T, Watt GC. Multimorbidity in primary care: Developing the research agenda. Fam Pract, 2009, 26(2), 79–80.

[41] Hannes K. Chapter 4: Critical appraisal of qualitative research. In: Noyes J, Booth A, Hannes K, Harden A, Harris J, Lewin S, eds. Supplementary guidance for inclusion of qualitative research in Cochrane systematic reviews of interventions. London, Cochrane Collaboration Qualitative Methods Group, 2011.

Sergej Kmetec, Zvonka Fekonja, Urša Markež,
Brendan McCormack, Urška Fekonja, Matej Strnad, Mateja Lorber

9 Triage of patients with acute coronary syndrome at the emergency department: a retrospective study

Abstract

Background: Acute coronary syndrome represents a considerable challenge worldwide as one of the causes of death; its diagnosis is often very complex. It includes acute myocardial infarction with ST-segment elevation, acute myocardial infarction without ST-segment elevation, unstable angina pectoris, and sudden cardiac arrest.

Methods: This retrospective cohort study included 678 patients who were admitted to the emergency department between 2015 and 2019 with acute coronary syndrome. Triage data were reviewed for vital signs, baseline characteristics, chief complaints, demographic variables, mode and time of arrival, triage, diagnosis, and treatment. Regression was used to identify key symptoms and patient characteristics at triage encounter to predict acute coronary syndrome.

Results: A total of 678 triage records were identified. The average age of the sample was 67 years old, 58.6% male, and 31.8% came by themselves to the emergency department. The most common diagnosis was acute myocardial infarctions without ST elevation (38.2%). Chest pain and difficulty in breathing were the two most common symptoms. Most patients were not assigned to the appropriate triage category, i.e., were diagnosed as less urgent.

Discussion and conclusion: This study presents the triage of patients with acute coronary syndrome at the emergency department to provide a comprehensive insight into their care. By identifying patient symptoms at the emergency department, nurse triage recognizes patients with acute coronary syndrome on time, thus increasing the accuracy of determining the triage category, which will impact the treatment outcome of patients.

Keywords: Acute myocardial infarction, Unstable angina pectoris, Heart arrest, Nurse, Triage

9.1 Introduction

Acute coronary symptom (ACS) represents a large healthcare problem worldwide, as one of the leading causes of death [1, 2]. It includes acute myocardial infarction with ST-segment elevation (STEMI), acute myocardial infarction (AMI) without ST-segment elevation (N-STEMI), and unstable angina pectoris (NAP) [3]. The cause in all forms of ACS is usually the same, and only the clinical presentation differs from one form to the other [3].

ACS occurs due to erosion or rupture of atherosclerotic coronary plaque where a blood clot forms, narrows, or closes the coronary lumen. In the area supplied by this artery, acute myocardial ischaemia develops. If ischaemia is severe and prolonged, this results in myocardial necrosis. The electric pulse conduction is also altered, which causes malignant ventricular tachyarrhythmia: ventricular tachycardia or fibrillation [4]. The occurrence of symptoms is often the first indicator of a change in health. Therefore, this can make it difficult for patients to identify accurately and interpret ACS symptoms on time, especially if the symptoms deviate from what the patient takes as a "normal state" or if the symptoms are like other non-cardiac ones [5]. Chest pain occurs at rest in 80% of ACS patients, and in the remaining 20% of patients at the slightest effort [6]. The pain is severe, burning, squeezing in the chest area, and extending into the neck, arms, and upper abdomen [7, 8]. Other accompanying symptoms include dyspnoea, nausea, vomiting, paleness, and perspiration [9].

It is important that triage nurses act quickly and, above all, correctly [10]. Rapid recognition of ACS symptoms is crucial for further treatment. Each triage nurse contributes to treating such a patient; therefore, it is important for them to be well-trained in the onset of ACS, the characteristic signs and symptoms, treatment methods, and response to any changes in health condition [11, 12].

To recognize ACS, it is important to record an electrocardiogram (ECG) and measure blood pressure, heart rate, saturation, and blood drawn according to the scheme laid down for ACS. An intravenous cannula is inserted for as much flow as possible, usually into the left cubital vein [13]. In the case of AMI, the patient is prepared for emergency coronary angiography, saving valuable time for the intervention healthcare team [14].

Triage nurses often do not recognize or miscategorize a patient suspected of having ACS [13]. Sanders and Devon [15] and Weeks and Edna Jones [16] note and add that triage nurses do not identify approximately 45% of these cases. Moreover, Benjamin et al. [17] state that one out of five patients with ACS dies early in the event of symptoms. With an early diagnosis of ACS, 10–20% mortality can be reduced, and the correct assessment at triage encounter is important [16, 17]. The clinical presentation of symptoms of a potential ACS is complex, and it is difficult for the triage nurse to distinguish between those who recognize an ACS and those who rule it out [18].

An accurate cardiac triage decision depends on triage nurses' personal traits, knowledge, and experience. The triage nurse must have sufficient experience and knowledge [19] of the common ACS symptoms, to prevent delays in treatment and improve treatment outcomes.

An early and accurate triage of a patient with suspected ACS is important to prevent delays in treatment and treatment outcomes [13]. Proper triage by the triage nurse leads to the fast taking of short anamnestic history, which is very important for further treatment, as survival, and later, the quality of the patient's life depend on it [14]. Triage nurses should be aware of all important patient symptoms and factors independently predictive of ACS.

The chapter aims to identify the demographic and other patient characteristics with ACS triaging by the triage nurse and present the treatment of patients with ACS in the emergency department (ED).

9.2 Methods

This study was based on the retrospective cohort study using multiple pre-existing data sources.

9.2.1 Setting

The study was conducted at a large medical centre's ED in Slovenia. Patient treatment data were obtained using pre-existing data sources in the medical records of patients. The records of all patients diagnosed with ACS were retrieved using a predetermined table and collected from 1 January 2015 to 31 December 2019.

9.2.2 Study population

This retrospective cohort study included medical records of adult patients (≥ 19 years), with the final diagnosis of ACS and its related diagnoses determined by the physician at discharge from ED or relocation to the ward. The exclusion criteria were medical records of younger patients (≤ 19 years) without a diagnosis of ACS and their related diagnoses determined by the physician at discharge from ED or relocation to the ward. Also, patient medical records with missing data, without Manchester Triage System (MTS), or unreadable font were excluded. Figure 9.1 displays the selection process of the medical record of patients with ACS.

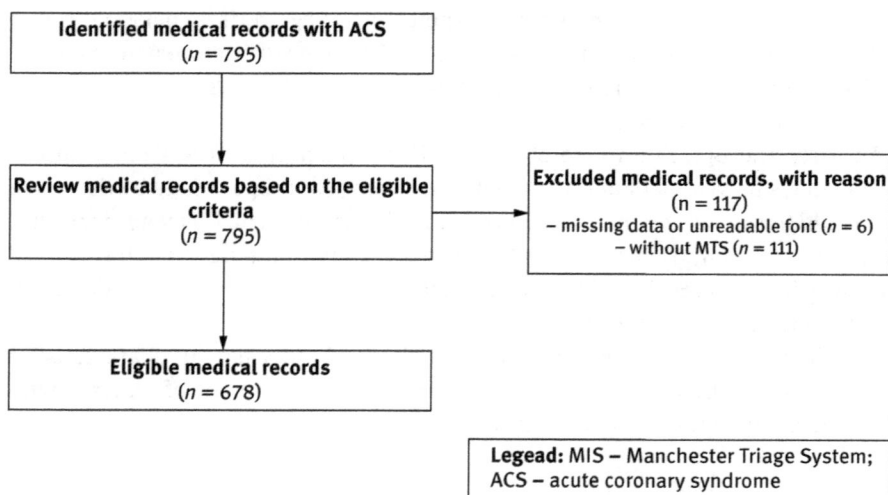

Fig. 9.1: The selection process of a patient's medical record with ACS. MTS, Manchester Triage System; ACS, acute coronary syndrome.

9.2.3 Statistical analysis

All data collected for this study were entered into a Microsoft Excel 2016 program and analysed using the SPSS 28.0 statistical program. Descriptive statistics were used to summarize and analyse the following information: demographic variables; mode and time of arrival; triage category; main problems; or cause for visiting the ED; diagnosis; treatment; and treatment outcome. The data were tested beforehand for normality, using the Shapiro–Wilk test. Based on the Shapiro–Wilk test, the data were not normally distributed ($W(678) = 0.649$, $p < 0.001$). The differences between the genders were tested with the Chi-square test, Mann–Whitney U test, and Kruskal–Wallis test, based on the variable type. Data were displayed as numbers on total (percentage), mean (M), and standard deviation (SD). Predictor variables were determined by univariate logistic regression (forward method, logit function, 95% confidence interval, $\alpha < 0.05$). The regression model fit was assessed by Pearson and Hosmer-Lemeshow tests. The sensitivity and specificity of the model were assessed by analysing the area under the ROC (receiver operating characteristic) curve, taking into account acceptable discrimination of $0.7 \leq \text{ROC} < 0.8$ [20]. The correlations between the values were verified by the Spearman correlation coefficient, considering: 0–0.09 (negligible), 0.10–0.39 (weak), 0.40–0.69 (moderate), 0.70–0.89, and 0.90–1 (very strong) [21]; $p \leq 0.05$ was considered statistically significant.

9.2.4 Ethical aspects

The study was approved by the Slovenian National Medical Ethics Committee (0120-69/2019/6) and received authorization from the selected institution. The study is retrospective, meaning that it includes patients who had already completed their treatment, and the study did not have an impact on the course of treatment. Data were analysed anonymously. The study followed the principles of the Declaration of Helsinki on Medical Research Involving Human Subjects [22] and the provisions of the Convention for the Protection of Human Rights and Dignity of the Human Being concerning the Application of Biology and Medicine (Oviedo Convention) [23].

9.3 Results

During the study period, 678 patients were treated for ACS at this ED. Due to incomplete or unreadable data and lack of MTS on medical records of patients, we excluded 117 (Fig. 9.1). The mean age was 67 years (SD = 13.7), and 41.4% (n = 281) were female. Based on the comparison between gender and age groups, we found that there was a statistical difference between the two variables ($\chi^2(1)$ = 22.073, p < 0.001). Women had mean age of 70.98 years (SD = 13.15), and men had 64.22 years (SD = 13.4). Of 678 patients were, 49% (n = 332) diagnosed with STEMI, 38.2% (n = 259) with N-STEMI, 6.3% (n = 43) with AP, and 6.5% (n = 44) with NAP. The final diagnosis was ACS only in 152 (22.4%) patients; 605 patients (89.2%) underwent immediate revascularization in the coronary catheterization laboratory, 54 patients (8%) were scheduled for coronary artery bypass surgery, 12 patients (1.8%) underwent pacemaker implantation, and seven patients (1%) were treated conservatively, as they refused coronary angiography. The demographic and clinical characteristics of the study population are presented in Tab. 9.1.

The overall mean systolic blood pressure was 154.24 mmHg (SD = 29.09) for the vital signs measured −156.07 mmHg (SD = 30.69) for women and 152.87 mmHg (SD = 28.10) for men. In terms of diastolic blood pressure, the overall mean was 87.93 mmHg (SD = 7.06), with 86.49 mmHg (SD = 16.37) in women and 88.94 mmHg (SD = 17.36) in men. The mean pulse rate for all patients was 83.54 beats/min (SD = 20.73). Only a statistical difference between sexes and pulse rate was found (Z = −2.175, p = 0.030). Women had a higher pulse rate on average (M = 85.58, SD = 20.79) than men (M = 81.89, SD = 20.49).

The treated patients came to the ED by different modes of arrival; 268 patients (39.5%) were brought by paramedics; 410 patients (60.5%) came from home by themselves, of which 214 (31.7%) patients were unaccompanied, and 464 (68.4%) patients were accompanied.

Tab. 9.1: Demographic and clinical characteristics.

Variable	DS	Gender ($n = 678$)		
		Male ($n = 397$)	Female ($n = 281$)	Z, χ^2 or r-value $\quad$ p
Age (Y; M ± SD; R)	67.02 ± 13.7; 20–94	64.22 ± 13.43; 20–92	70.98 ± 13.15; 25–94	
<65 years	299(44.1)	205(51.6)	94(33.5)	22,073[a] <0.001*
≥65 years	379(60)	192(48.4)	187(66.5)	
Vital signs				
SBP** (M ± SD)	154.24 ± 29.09	152.87 ± 28.10	156.07 ± 30.69	−1.424[b] 0.154
DBP** (M ± SD)	87.93 ± 17.06	88.94 ± 17.36	86.49 ± 16.37	−1.552[b] 0.121
Pulse (M ± SD)	83.54 ± 20.73	81.89 ± 20.49	85.58 ± 20.79	−2.175[b] 0.030*
SpO$_2$ (M ± SD)	95.54 ± 3.99	95.84 ± 3.68	95.85 ± 0.90	−0.211[b] 0.833
Triage MTS (M ± SD)	2.78 ± 0.70; 2–4	2.74 ± 0.71	2.85 ± 0.69	
Red n(%)	0(0)	0(0)	0(0)	5.599[a] 0.061
Orange n(%)	255(37.6)	164(41.3)	91(32.4)	
Yellow n(%)	315(46.5)	173(43.6)	142(50.5)	
Green n(%)	108(15.9)	60(15.1)	48(17.1)	
Blue n(%)	0(0)	0(0)	0(0)	
Type of ASC n(%)	678(100)			
STEMI, n(%)	332(49)	191(48.1)	141(50.2)	0.422[c] 0.516
N-STEMI, n(%)	259(38.2)	153(38.5)	106(37.7)	
NAP, n(%)	44(6.5)	24(6)	20(7.1)	
AP, n(%)	43(6.3)	29(7.3)	14(5)	
Number of symptoms (M ± SD, R)	2.5 ± 1.19; 1–6	2.39 ± 1.17; 1–6	2.67 ± 1.18; 1–6	−3.418[b] 0.001*

*, Statistical significance ($p < 0.05$); **, mmHg; %, per cent of participants; a, Chi-square test; AP, angina pectoris; b, Mann–Whitney U test; c, Kruskal–Wallis test; DS, descriptive statistics; M, mean; MTS, Manchester Triage System; n, sample size; N-STEMI, non-ST elevation myocardial infarction; NAP, unstable angina pectoris; SD, standard deviation; STEMI, ST-elevation myocardial infarction.

The patients requiring help at the ED who delayed their problems for a few hours numbered 323 (47.6%), 131 patients (19.3%) delayed their problems for a while, 84 patients (12.4%) sought help within a few minutes after the onset of health problems, 63 patients (9.3%) within 10 min, and most of the patients within 30 min ($n = 77$, 11.4%). There were 194 patients (18.6%) who arrived within a few hours (≤ 6 h), of which most arrived within 1 h ($n = 84$, 12.4%) (Tab. 9.2).

Tab. 9.2: Duration of symptoms ($n = 678$).

Variable	n(%)
0–1 h	84(12.4)
1–6 h	110(16.2)
6–12 h	17(2.5)
12–24 h	79(11.7)
More than 24 h	388(52.2)

%, per cent of participants; n, sample size.

All patients were triaged into triage categories by colour: the orange triage category, in which patients must be provided medical assistance within 10 min, was assigned to 255 patients (37.6%), and the yellow triage category, which also represents the largest group of treated patients requiring medical assistance within 60 min, was assigned to 315 patients (46.5%), and the green triage category, where patients wait up to 120 min for treatment, was assigned to 108 patients (15.9%) (see Tab. 9.1). The most common triage algorithm selected by the Registered Nurse was chest pain (45.9%), adult malaise (17.7%), and dyspnoea (6.5%). The most common triage criteria chosen for triage were moderate pain (10.6%), recent problems (10.3%), rapid onset (7.9%), angina pectoris (7.6%), history of significant heart disease (6.3%), pleuritic pain (4.6%), and low SpO_2 (4.3%).

We observed significant difference between mean MTS levels concerning the most common symptoms (chest pain: 2.75 ± 0.69, shortness of breath: 2.81 ± 0.73, nausea: 2.96 ± 0.79, pain in the left arm: 2.81 ± 0.60, $p < 0.001$) and type of ACS (STEMI: 2.76 ± 0.70; N-STEMI: 2.79 ± 0.70; and NAP: 2.70 ± 0.69, AP: 3.00 ± 0.72, $p < 0.001$). There was no significant difference in gender (male: 2.74 ± 0.71, female: 2.85 ± 0.69, $p = 0.061$), age groups (age < 65 years: 2.78 ± 0.70, age ≥ 65 years: 2.79 ± 0.70, $p = 0.990$), and concerning diabetes (diabetic: 2.81 ± 0.69, non-diabetic: $2.78 \pm .70$, $p = 0.763$) (Tab. 9.3).

Patients reported a mean of 2.5 symptoms (SD = 1.19). The most common symptoms provided by the patient, which are more likely to lead to the development of ACS, were chest pain ($n = 568$, 83.8%), difficult breathing ($n = 192$, 28.3%), nausea ($n = 99$, 14.6%), pain in the left arm ($n = 74$, 10.9%), sweating ($n = 67$, 9.9%), dizziness

Tab. 9.3: Average MTS levels with a standard deviation of the study sample.

Variables	Mean MTS level ± SD	p
All (n = 678)		
Men	2.74 ± 0.71	0.061
Women	2.85 ± 0.69	
Age < 65 years	2.78 ± 0.70	0.990
Age ≥ 65 years	2.79 ± 0.70	
Chest pain	2.75 ± 0.69	<0.001*
Shortness of breath	2.81 ± 0.73	
Nausea	2.96 ± 0.79	
Pain in the left arm	2.81 ± 0.60	
Diabetes	2.81 ± 0.69	0.763
No diabetes	2.78 ± 0.70	
STEMI	2.76 ± 0.70	<0.001*
N-STEMI	2.79 ± 0.70	
NAP	2.70 ± 0.69	
AP	3.00 ± 0.72	

*, Statistical significance at $p < 0.05$; AP, angina pectoris; MTS, Manchester Triage System; N-STEMI, non-ST elevation myocardial infarction; NAP, Unstable angina pectoris; SD, standard deviation; STEMI, ST elevation myocardial infarction.

(n = 52, 7.7%), pain on exertion (n = 47, 6.9%), general weakness (n = 45, 6.6%), and vomiting (n = 43, 6.3%). Other medical histories were atypical for ACS and occurred in less than 5% of patients.

All 678 (100%) patients had ECG performed, and 677 patients (99.9%) had blood drawn according to the ACS regimen. Other examinations performed on patients included X-rays (n = 62, 9.1%), laboratory urine tests (n = 4, 0.6%), and ultrasound of the lungs or heart (n = 5, 0.7%).

The most administered drug therapies at the ED prescribed by the physician during medical treatment were acetylsalicylic acid 250 mg (n = 341, 50.3%), glyceryl nitrate (n = 253, 37.3%), sodium chloride (n = 117, 17.3%), morphine (n = 83, 12.2%), and heparin (n = 64, 9.4%).

Among the associated diseases of the treated patients with ACS, the most common were arterial hypertension (n = 414, 61.1%), hyperlipidaemia (n = 180, 26.5%), diabetes type 2 (n = 144, 21.2%), and other diseases shown in Tab. 9.4.

Tab. 9.4: Patients' associated diseases.

Major adverse cardiac event risk factors	Men (*n* = 397)	Women (*n* = 281)	Total (*n* = 678)
	n(%)	*n*(%)	*n*(%)
Arterial hypertension	225(33.2)	189(27.9)	414(61.1)
Hyperlipidaemia	108(15.9)	72(10.6)	180(26.5)
Diabetes type 2	86(12.7)	58(8.6)	144(21.2)
Acute myocardial infarction	69(10.2)	29(4.3)	98(14.5)
Atrial fibrillation	37(5.5)	33(4.9)	70(10.3)
Heart failure	28(4.1)	34(5)	62(9.1)
Dyslipidaemia	34(5)	11(1.6)	45(6.6)
Chronic kidney disease	16(2.4)	26(3.8)	42(6.2)
Ischemic heart disease	22(3.2)	12(1.8)	34(5)
Angina pectoris	16(2.4)	14(2.1)	30(4.4)
Asthma	12(1.8)	15(2.2)	27(4)
Chronic obstructive pulmonary disease	17(2.5)	6(.9)	23(3.4)

%, per cent of participants; *n*, sample size.

Ninety-eight patients (14.5% of all patients) had already experienced AMI. One patient recovered from AMI three times, that is, 35, 29, and 22 years ago. Eight patients (1.2%) had AMI twice, the remaining patients (89 patients or 13.1%) had AMI once, and for 18 patients (2.7%), we did not obtain the year of AMI. Recurrent AMI is most common in the first few years after AMI. Cardiac arrest was experienced by 3 (0.4%) patients treated, that is, 3, 10, and 12 years ago.

Patients were hospitalized for a mean nine days (SD = 8.5). The longest hospitalization took 64 days (SD = 15.6), and the patient who was hospitalized the least was discharged on the same day he was admitted. Of all hospitalized patients, 32 patients (4.7%) died during the hospitalization. Only eight patients (1.2%) died due to ACS; in other patients (*n* = 24, 3.5%), the causes were congestive heart failure, cardiogenic shock, pneumonia, other types of shock, and others.

With Spearman's correlations (Tab. 9.5), we found negative correlations between chest pain and other symptoms of acute coronary syndrome – difficult breathing and chest pain ($r_s = -0.375$; $p < 0.01$), nausea and chest pain ($r_s = -0.312$; $p < 0.01$), and pain in the left arm and chest pain ($r_s = -0.199$; $p < 0.01$). Table 9.5 shows a further finding of a positive correlation between final diagnosis and duration of the symptoms ($r_s = 0.132$; $p < 0.01$) and final diagnosis and chest pain ($r_s = 0.134$; $p < 0.01$).

Tab. 9.5: Spearman correlation matrix of MTS, duration of symptoms, and most common symptoms of ACS.

Variable	MTS	Duration of symptoms	Chest pain	Difficult breathing	Nausea	Pain in the left arm
MTS	1	−0.061	−0.122	0.015*	0.108	−0.004*
Duration of symptoms	−0.061	1	0.214	−0.158	−0.047*	−0.026*
Chest pain	−0.122	0.214	1	−0.375	−0.312	−0.199
Difficult breathing	0.015*	−0.158	−0.375	1	−0.058*	−0.037*
Nausea	0.108	−0.047*	−0.312	−0.058*	1	−0.031*
Pain in the left arm	−0.004*	−0.026*	−0.199	−0.037*	−0.031*	1

*, Statistical significance at $p < 0.05$; MTS, Manchester Triage System.

Tab. 9.6: Regression results for the symptoms of ACS.

Variable	B	SE	β	t	p
Final diagnosis	−3.859	23.543	.229	−0.164	0.870
Duration of symptoms	4.038	1.217	0.129	3.317	0.001*
Triage colour	0.948	0.947	0.038	1.000	0.317
Chest pain	0.154	0.048	0.148	3.217	0.001*
Difficult breathing	0.034	0.086	0.017	0.398	0.691
Nausea	0.014	0.100	0.006	0.140	0.889
Pain in the left arm	0.295	0.149	0.077	1.979	0.048*
$R = 0.124$; adjusted $R^2 = 0.310$; SE = 1.922; $F = 2.635$ ($p < 0.001$)					

*, Statistical significance at $p < 0.05$; B, estimated values of raw (unstandardized) regression coefficient; F, F distribution; n, sample size; p, probability; R, unstandardized regression coefficient; R^2, unstandardized regression squared coefficient; SE, standard error; t, Student's t distribution; and β, beta coefficient.

The data show that the overall regression was statistically significant ($R^2 = 0.124$, $F(4.635) = 2.635$, $p < 0.001$). Concerning the value of the standardized regression coefficient among the studied variables, we found that the duration of symptoms ($\beta = 0.129$; $p < 0.001$) has the strongest impact on chest pain ($\beta = 0.148$ $p < 0.001$), followed by the triage colour ($\beta = 0.038$, $p = 0.317$), difficult breathing ($\beta = 0.017$; $p = 0.691$), pain in the left arm ($\beta = 0.077$; $p = 0.048$), and nausea ($\beta = 0.06$; $p = 0.889$). The multiple regression analysis showed that we can explain 31% of the total variability of most prevalent symptoms of patients that lead to serious cardiac diseases, the duration of symptoms, chest pain, and pain in the left arm (Tab. 9.6).

9.4 Discussion

We present the treatment of patients with ACS at the ED, demonstrating the complexity of the highlighted issue. The mean age of the patients with ACS was 67 years, 58.6% male, and 31.8% came by themselves to the ED. The most common diagnosis was AMI without ST elevation (38.2%). Among the associated diseases of the treated patients with ACS, the most common was arterial hypertension. Chest pain and difficult breathing were the two most common symptoms as a reason for seeking help at the ED. Most patients were not assigned to the appropriate triage category, i.e., were diagnosed as less urgent. Most patients had ECG performed, and blood was drawn according to the ACS regimen. Other examinations performed on patients included X–rays, laboratory urine tests, and ultrasounds of the lungs or heart.

This chapter also identifies key symptoms and factors in patients that were available to triage nurses in the initial assessment of an ED patient's health status. The final model showed that the following baseline predictors have good differentiating value for ACS detection during initial nursing triage: chest pain, duration of symptoms, and left arm pain. By knowing which patient factors are important when a patient enters an ED seeking emergency care, triage nurses can prioritize treatment and provide timely care to those most in need of adequate ED resources, greatly impacting outcomes in ACS populations. The complexity of ACS requires much knowledge about this condition and its occurrence to identify, take measures, and treat such patients promptly, as timely and quality treatment of patients with ACS is very important. Recognizing clinical signs of ACS begins with the patient's admission at triage encounter, which was continuously performed at the ED.

In the United States, more than 5.5 million patients with symptoms suspected of ACS come to the emergency every year [18], of which 20–25% have a final diagnosis of ACS [24], while in Slovenia, this number is around 5,000 people annually [9]. In this study, 197,456 people required medical assistance, of which 678 patients who sought help in the ED had ACS diagnosed.

Triage nurses should be aware of all underlying conditions of patient factors that independently predict ACS [13]. Identifying the patient's ACS factors in the first minutes of triage is important in determining the most predictable symptoms of ACS. Approximately one in five patients with ACS will die very early in treatment [17]. According to Benjamin et al. [17] and Wu et al. [25], making an early diagnosis of ACS can reduce mortality by 10–20%. Eisen et al. [26] and Sinkovič [27] report that the prevalence of N-STEMI is certainly much higher than for other ACS conditions, as well as NAP. Moreover, STEMI, on the other hand, accounts for only a third of all ACS conditions. STEMI (49% of all treated patients) was the most diagnosed at the ED, followed by N-STEMI (38.2%), AP (6.3%), and NAP (6.5%). Of all patients treated, 58.6% were men, and 41.4% were women. Different studies [28–30] also found that the prevalence of ACS is higher in men than in women at different ages. The mean age of the treated patients was 67 years (SD = 13.7), suggesting that the prevalence of ACS is higher in older than in younger patients [29]. In our study, the oldest patients were born in 1923, and the youngest was born in 1996. The most common symptoms in almost all treated patients included chest pain, followed by shortness of breath. According to Gillis et al. [31], chest pain and shortness of breath are the most common symptoms in the elderly, which can also be confirmed in our study.

Patients in our study reported a mean of three symptoms (SD = 1.2); however, the study conducted by Kirchberger et al. [32] reports 4.6 symptoms: most commonly, diaphoresis (61%), left shoulder and arm pain (56.7%), and dyspnoea (48.5%). Furthermore, the study showed that patients with STEMI reported significantly more symptoms than patients with N-STEMI. Our study also found that patients with STEMI reported a mean of 2.6 symptoms (SD = 1.2), and patients with N-STEMI reported 2.4 symptoms (SD = 1.3). Patients who experienced vomiting, diaphoresis, or dizziness were found to have a significantly higher risk of developing STEMI. In contrast, dyspnoea and neck pain were associated with an increased risk of N-STEMI.

STEMI was the most commonly diagnosed among the ACS, and chest pain as a symptom was present in most patients. Due to the increasing number of patient visits to ED, triage is becoming more important in ED to prioritize and treat patients with potentially life-threatening diseases such as ACS [33]. According to the MTS, patients with ACS should be classified into red and orange categories [34]. Our retrospective study demonstrates that patients diagnosed with ACS were triaged as MTS level 2 and MTS level 3 (very urgent to urgent assessment) and should be seen by the physician within 10–60 min. After reviewing the triage records, we found that no patients were classified in the red category, which can be explained by the direct admission of those patients to the treatment beyond triage. Only a quarter of all triage patients were classified in the appropriate orange category. This means that the remaining treated patients were assigned to an inappropriate or lower triage category than they should be. International research suggests that many patients (even more than 50%) with ACS are classified into lower triage categories than they should otherwise be [35]. Chest pain was absent in as many as 21.6% of patients in this category, resulting from the selected lower triage category, and N-STEMI was the most frequently diagnosed in this category.

In this chapter, we present the treatment of a patient with ACS at the ED, demonstrating the complexity of the highlighted issue. The study may be helpful to all healthcare professionals who perform their work at the ED and provides insight into the treatment of these patients. Continuous education of employees is very important, as we established in the study how difficult it is to recognize ACS due to many factors and the occurrence of unusual symptoms. According to many authors [17, 36], the prevalence of ACS is certainly growing; therefore, educating the patients and the general population to take preventive interventions is necessary.

Our study does not provide insight into the actual situation or the number of treated patients, as we recorded only those who sought help at the selected ED and had a final diagnosis of ACS. We also gained insight into only one ED, so it would make sense to investigate the prevalence of ACS elsewhere in Slovenia, in a larger sample and include a prehospital unit. Many authors also report the delayed time to primary percutaneous intervention as the cause of treatment complications during hospitalization and high mortality, so it would be sensible to record the average time until intervention and determine whether this time is approximately the same as the duration recommended by international guidelines.

9.5 Conclusion

The population is ageing, and increasingly, people have various associated chronic diseases and unhealthy lifestyles, which increases the possibility of developing ACS that is difficult to identify in older patients. Timely diagnosis and treatment of ACS are crucial for the prognosis of the disease and the quality of the patient's subsequent life. Symptoms with good distinctive value have been found to identify patients with potential ACS at triage. These key patient symptoms need to be considered in the initial health assessment and can help triage nurses better differentiate patients with symptoms suggestive of ACS, and help provide faster care to those in need of immediate treatment. Therefore, the work of a triage nurse is extremely important in the triage encounter, as it depends on her/him, if the most threatening symptoms to the patient are recognized in time and treated promptly.

References

[1]   World Health Organization. Noncommunicable diseases progress monitor 2020. Geneva, World Health Organization, 2020.
[2]   Condén E, Rosenblad A, Wagner P, Leppert J, Ekselius L, Åslund C. Is type D personality an independent risk factor for recurrent myocardial infarction or all-cause mortality in post-acute myocardial infarction patients? Eur J Prev Cardiol, 2020, 24(5), 522–533.
[3]   Davis LL, Maness JJ. Nurse practitioner knowledge of symptoms of acute coronary syndrome. J Nurs Pract, 2019, 15(1), e9–e12.
[4]   Tkacs N, Herrmann L, Johnson R. Advanced physiology and pathophysiology: Essentials for clinical practice. Springer Publishing Company, 2020.
[5]   Mehilli J, Presbitero P. Coronary artery disease and acute coronary syndrome in women. Heart, 2020, 106(7), 487–492.
[6]   Haider A, Bengs S, Luu J, Osto E, Siller-Matula JM, Muka T, et al. Sex and gender in cardiovascular medicine: Presentation and outcomes of acute coronary syndrome. Eur Heart J, 2020, 41(13), 1328–1336.
[7]   De Leon K, Winokur EJ. Examining acute coronary syndrome across ethnicity, sex, and age. J Nurs Pract, 2022, 18(1), 31–35.
[8]   DeVon HA, Mirzaei S, Zègre-Hemsey J. Typical and atypical symptoms of acute coronary syndrome: Time to retire the terms? J Am Heart Assoc, 2020, 9(7), e015539.

[9] Radšel P, Čerček M, Lipar L, Kompara G, Prosen G, Noč M. Akutni koronarni sindrom: Smernice za obravnavo v Sloveniji v letu 2015. Ljubljana, Društvo Iatros, društvo za napredek v medicini, 2015.

[10] Bijani M, Khaleghi AA. Challenges and barriers affecting the quality of triage in emergency departments: A qualitative study. Galen Med J, 2019, 8, e1619.

[11] Zhiting G, Jingfen J, Shuihong C, Minfei Y, Yuwei W, Sa W. Reliability and validity of the four-level Chinese emergency triage scale in mainland China: A multicentre assessment. Int J Nurs Stud, 2020, 101, 103447.

[12] King-Shier K, Quan H, Kapral MK, Tsuyuki R, An L, Banerjee S, et al. Acute coronary syndromes presentations and care outcomes in white, South Asian and Chinese patients: A cohort study. BMJ Open, 2019, 9(3), e022479.

[13] Frisch SO, Brown J, Faramand Z, Stemler J, Sejdić E, Martin-Gill C, et al. Exploring the complex interactions of baseline patient factors to improve nursing triage of acute coronary syndrome. Res Nurs Health, 2020, 43(4), 356–364.

[14] Miložič L, Lešnik A. The work and role of a nurse at internal medicine emergency room with patients with acute myocardial infarction. In: Rajko V, Gričar M, eds. Emergency medicine: Selected topics: Proceedings. Ljubljana, Slovenian Society for Emergency Medicine, 2015, 300–303.

[15] Sanders SF, DeVon HA. Accuracy in ED triage for symptoms of acute myocardial infarction. J Emerg Nurs, 2016, 42(4), 331–337.

[16] Weeks J, Edna Jones M. Are triage nurse knowledgeable about acute coronary syndromes recognition? ABNF J, 2017, 28(3), 69–75.

[17] Benjamin EJ, Virani SS, Callaway CW, Chamberlain AM, Chang AR, Cheng S, et al. Heart disease and stroke statistics-2018 update: A report from the American heart association. Circulation, 2018, 137(12), e67–e492.

[18] Mirzaei S, Steffen A, Vuckovic K, Ryan C, Bronas U, Zegre-Hemsey J, et al. The quality of symptoms in women and men presenting to the emergency department with suspected acute coronary syndrome. J Emerg Nurs, 2019, 45(4), 357–365.

[19] Burström L, Letterstål A, Engström ML, Berglund A, Enlund M. The patient safety culture as perceived by staff at two different emergency departments before and after introducing a flow-oriented working model with team triage and lean principles: A repeated cross-sectional study. BMC Health Serv Res, 2014, 14, 296.

[20] Lopes AR, Nihei OK. Burnout among nursing students: Predictors and association with empathy and self-efficacy. Rev Bras Enferm, 2020, 73(1), e20180280.

[21] Schober P, Boer C, Schwarte LA. Correlation coefficients: Appropriate use and interpretation. Anesth Analg, 2018, 126(5), 1763–1768.

[22] World Medical Association. Declaration of Helsinki. Ethical principles for medical research involving human subjects. Jahrbuch Für Wissenschaft Und Ethik, 2009, 14(1), 233–238.

[23] Council of Europe. Convention for the protection of human rights and dignity of the human being with regard to the application of biology and medicine (European tratyseries-no. 164). Oviedo, Council of Europe.

[24] Kumar A, Cannon CP. Acute coronary syndromes: Diagnosis and management, part I. Mayo Clin Proc, 2009, 84(10), 917–938.

[25] Wu J, Gale CP, Hall M, Dondo TB, Metcalfe E, Oliver G, et al. Editor's Choice – Impact of initial hospital diagnosis on mortality for acute myocardial infarction: A national cohort study. Eur Heart J Acute Cardiovasc Care, 2018, 7(2), 139–148.

[26] Eisen A, Giugliano RP, Braunwald E. Updates on acute coronary syndrome: A review. JAMA Cardiol, 2016, 1(6), 718–730.

[27]   Sinkovič A. Akutni koronarni sindrom (AKS) – opredelitev, patogeneza, ocena tveganja,
        obravnava. In: Grosek Š, Podbregar M, Gradišek P, eds. Šola intenzivne medicine: 2 letnik:
        Endokrinologija, koagulacija, akutni koronarni sindrom z ostalimi srčnimi boleznimi in
        bolezni respiracijskega sistema: Učbenik. Ljubljana, Slovensko združenje za intenzivno
        medicino, 2014, 131–134.
[28]   Duan JG, Chen XY, Wang L, Lau A, Wong A, Thomas GN, et al. Sex differences in epidemiology
        and risk factors of acute coronary syndrome in Chinese patients with type 2 diabetes: A long-
        term prospective cohort study. PLOS ONE, 2015, 10(4), e0122031.
[29]   Ekelund U, Akbarzadeh M, Khoshnood A, Björk J, Ohlsson M. Likelihood of acute coronary
        syndrome in emergency department chest pain patients varies with time of presentation.
        BMC Res Notes, 2012, 5(1), 420.
[30]   Sanchis-Gomar F, Perez-Quilis C, Leischik R, Lucia A. Epidemiology of coronary heart disease
        and acute coronary syndrome. Ann Transl Med, 2016, 4(13), 256.
[31]   Gillis NK, Arslanian-Engoren C, Struble LM. Acute coronary syndromes in older adults:
        A review of literature. J Emerg Nurs, 2014, 40(3), 270–275. quiz 92.
[32]   Kirchberger I, Meisinger C, Heier M, Kling B, Wende R, Greschik C, et al. Patient-reported
        symptoms in acute myocardial infarction: Differences related to ST-segment elevation: The
        MONICA/KORA myocardial infarction registry. J Intern Med, 2011, 270(1), 58–64.
[33]   Kiblboeck D, Steinrueck K, Nitsche C, Lang W, Kellermair J, Blessberger H, et al. Evaluation of
        the Manchester triage system for patients with acute coronary syndrome. Wien Klin
        Wochenschr, 2020, 132(11–12), 277–282.
[34]   Nishi FA, Maia F, de Souza Santos I. Assessing sensitivity and specificity of the Manchester
        triage system in the evaluation of acute coronary syndrome in adult patients in emergency
        care: A systematic review. JBI Evidence Synthesis, 2017, 15(6), 1747–1761.
[35]   Ryan K, Greenslade J, Dalton E, Chu K, Brown AF, Cullen L. Factors associated with triage
        assignment of emergency department patients ultimately diagnosed with acute myocardial
        infarction. Aust Crit Care, 2016, 29(1), 23–26.
[36]   Rodríguez-Mañero M, Cordero A, Kreidieh O, García-Acuña JM, Seijas J, Agra-Bermejo RM,
        et al. Proposal of a novel clinical score to predict heart failure incidence in long-term
        survivors of acute coronary syndromes. Int J Cardiol, 2017, 249, 301–307.

Sergej Kmetec, Zvonka Fekonja, Vida Gönc, Brendan McCormack

10 Palliative care for patients with heart failure: a cross-sectional study among nursing healthcare professionals

Abstract

Background: Acute heart failure is a problem that the public healthcare system faces worldwide. Despite improving healthcare systems and the resulting treatment, the disease's incidence and frequency has increased annually. Therefore, patients with acute heart failure often seek help in the emergency room, where nursing health professionals encounter the condition early or late. In the final stages, they need to focus on providing palliative care to such patients. The chapter aims to determine the nursing healthcare professionals' knowledge, perceptions, and attitudes towards palliative care in patients with heart failure in the emergency and cardiology departments.

Methods: A cross-sectional study was carried out. The survey took place in August 2019 involving nursing healthcare professionals.

Results: Of 104 nurses, 50% ($n = 52$) had received training in palliative care throughout their education and 7.7% ($n = 8$) had received additional training. Nursing healthcare professionals in both the emergency and the cardiology departments have similar knowledge about palliative care. With regard to the perception of implementing palliative care, the data shows a statistically significant difference between both departments. Furthermore, statistically significant differences between the emergency and cardiology departments have been found in some statements regarding their attitudes, namely that there remains a need for palliative care in treating patients with heart failure.

Discussion and conclusion: We believe that the knowledge of palliative care in the cardiology and emergency departments is good, and that there are no major differences between the knowledge and departments. However, further training is required to improve the healthcare staff's knowledge, perceptions, and attitudes towards palliative care in patients with heart failure.

Keywords: acute heart failure chronic heart failure palliative care attitudes knowledge perceived obstacles nurse

10.1 Introduction

Heart failure is a global public health problem [1], characterized by high mortality rates, increased emergency visits, hospital admissions and readmissions, and a massive economic burden on the national health systems [2, 3]. Among cardiovascular diseases, heart failure is the only one whose incidence and prevalence increases annually [4] with increasing age, despite advances in risk factor control and better pharmacological treatments [5]. Approximately 26 million people worldwide are diagnosed with heart failure; 2 million are diagnosed newly each year, with survival estimates of roughly 10% after ten years of diagnosis [6–8]. Epidemical data shows that 6.5 million people in Europe, 5 million people in the United States of America [9] and 2.4 million people in Japan have heart failure [7]. Acute exacerbation of chronic heart failure is one of the most common reasons for emergency department (ED) visits [10]. Worldwide, the ED represents an important entry point for treating such patients [11]. Patients with acute heart failure presenting to the ED have different symptoms, such as dyspnoea, depression, pain, fatigue, shortness of breath and peripheral oedema [1, 11, 12]. Other manifestations such as hypotension, dizziness and bradycardia may also occur [1]. After the initial stabilization of the condition, one of the most important decisions is to determine which patients can be safely discharged home and which should be hospitalized. Taking such a complex decision depends on several subjective factors, including the severity of the patient's underlying health condition [13].

ED nursing healthcare professionals often encounter early- and end-stage heart failure patients where the disease is no longer curable, and their focus shifts from curative treatment to palliative care [14]. Palliative care includes symptom assessment and treatment, help with decision-making and setting goals of care, practical support for patients and care partners, mobilizing community support and resources to provide a safe and secure living environment, and focusing on relieving the distress of symptoms. Here, transdisciplinary palliative care teams can help with complex medical decision-making about life-sustaining treatments and facilitate alternative discharge plans [15].

Although not considered ideal to start palliative care in the ED, it is the most frequented and dynamic environment. Whether there are gaps in the outpatient setting or a failure to anticipate and plan for crisis intervention, the ED experience can be crucial in determining the patient's pathway. The ED culture of stabilizing acute medical emergencies is shifting to a more focused culture of person-centred palliative care [9] –early detection, assessment and treatment of pain and other physical, psychosocial and other problems – reducing symptom burden and improving the quality of life [16]. Although the emergency room represents a common point of contact for patients with life-threatening diseases, nursing healthcare professionals must be able to recognize the need to provide general palliative care [17]. According to Sanad [18], palliative care is not the prevailing mindset of emergency healthcare teams, as they consider this type of care to be outside their scope of practice or even contrary to the principles of emergency medicine [19–23]. The need for collaboration between trans-disciplinary palliative care and emergency healthcare teams has been recognized in various studies [19, 20, 24]. Moreover, the authors, Ieraci [19], Lukin et al. [25] and Todd [24], conclude that attitudes and knowledge about palliative care represent potential barriers to the identification and implementation of such an approach [17]. Therefore, the knowledge, perceptions, and attitudes of both emergency healthcare teams and cardiology healthcare teams regarding palliative care and their perceived role are important to improve the emergency and cardiology departments in implementing such an approach [18]. Some evidence is available regarding palliative care for heart failure patients [26, 27]. However, there is a gap in the management of palliative care of patients with heart failure in the ED where such treatment should start and follow up in the cardiology department. For optimal palliative care for heart failure, nursing healthcare professionals should receive adequate training in providing palliative care in the ED and cardiology departments. Nursing healthcare professionals can improve the quality of life of patients with heart failure who have been discharged to home care or tertiary care by applying the principles of palliative care. The chapter aims, therefore, to determine nursing healthcare professionals' knowledge, perceptions, and attitudes towards palliative care in patients with heart failure in the ED and cardiology departments.

10.2 Methods

10.2.1 Study design

The study used a cross-sectional design applied using a paper-based questionnaire. This study involved looking at data from a population viewpoint at a specific time. Participants were selected based on certain variables of interest. Cross-sectional studies are observational and known as descriptive research, not causal or relational. The researcher cannot use a survey to determine the cause of something such as a disease [28]. To ensure the adequate and complete reporting of the study, we followed the STROBE guidelines [29].

10.2.2 Settings and participants

The study was carried out in one ED and one cardiology department that offered regional secondary care for patients with heart failure in the Styria region of Slovenia. This study recruited a convenience sample of nursing healthcare professionals with a high school (secondary education), or first-, second-, or third-level Bologna degree. In addition, the inclusion criteria included nursing healthcare professionals with at least 12 months of work experience in the ED or cardiology department. The exclusion criteria were nursing healthcare professionals who did not have a high school (second-ary education), or first, second or third level Bologna degree in nursing and/or did not work for at least 12 months in the ED or cardiology departments. When carried out, all nursing healthcare professionals on duty were invited to participate in the survey. Be-fore collecting the questionnaires, the sample size represented was calculated accord-ing to the Cochran formula [30]. The results of the procedure showed a minimum number of 103 participants, considering the following parameters: n (the sample size), z (confidence level – 95%), p (the estimated proportion of the attribute present in the population), $q = 1-p$, and e (the desired level of precision at ±5%).

10.2.3 Data collection and measures

A questionnaire that was validated by Ziehm et al. [16] was used to obtain data. The questionnaire consists of two sections. The first section relates to demographic informa-tion (e. g., gender, age, education, and work experience). The second section of the questionnaire consists of six sets of sub-questions ($n = 72$). The first part of the statement relates to knowledge of the definition of palliative care and expectations regarding the provision of palliative care. The second part of the statement refers to the organizational conditions for implementing palliative care. The third part covers the barriers encoun-tered by patients with heart failure. The fourth part concerns the determination of the usefulness of palliative care. The fifth part contains statements about the appropriate time to start palliative care for the patient. In the final part, the nursing care professio-nals were asked if they could distinguish between general and specialized palliative care. The items could be answered on a 5-point Likert scale (from 1 = "strongly agree" to 5 = "strongly disagree"). Two questions stated that answers could be "yes" or "no".

The content validity of the questionnaire was guided by Polit and Beck's [28] guidelines. We also checked the appropriateness of the questionnaire structure, ap-pearance, feasibility, readability, consistency of style between questions, formatting, and clarity of language. Ten experts who had worked in palliative care and the divi-sion of internal medicine for more than five years were intentionally chosen. Minor changes were made to the questions based on the review, and the expert panel sub-sequently approved the questionnaire. The questionnaire was pilot–tested with a small sample of healthcare professionals ($n = 75$) to assess its reliability using Cron-bach's alpha. The Cronbach's alpha of the questionnaire was excellent ($\alpha = 0.923$).

The survey took place in August 2019. Based on the required sample size of 103 nursing healthcare professionals and the estimated response rate, 180 question-naires were distributed. Questionnaires were distributed in paper form with the as-sistance of head nurses of each department, and the completed questionnaires were returned in a sealed envelope. One hundred and fifty-two questionnaires were returned, some partially completed (half of the answers were missing, while the response rate was 68.4%). Forty-eight questionnaires were excluded based on a 50% non-completion rate, and the final sample size of the survey was 104.

10.2.4 Data analysis

Data were imported and analysed using SPSS IBM version 28. Descriptive and inferential statistics were used to analyze the results. Data was displayed as numbers on total (percentage), mean (M), and standard deviation (SD). Beforehand, the data was tested for normality using the Shapiro–Wilk test. Since the data were not normally distributed ($W(104) = .569$, $p <0.001$), the differences in knowledge, perceptions, and attitudes towards palliative care between the ED and cardiology departments were tested with the Mann–Whitney U-test. The correlations between the work experience and attitudes of the nursing healthcare professionals towards providing palliative care to patients with heart failure were verified by the Spearman correlation coefficient, considering: <0.09 (negligible), 0.10–0.39 (weak), 0.40–0.69 (moderate), 0.70–0.89 (strong) and 0.90–1.0 (very strong) [31]. A statistical significance of the results was considered if p-values were less than 0.05 [28].

10.2.5 Ethical approval

Ethical approval was obtained before we conducted the study (ref. no.: 038/2019/5341-2/504) and received authorization from the selected institution. Participants were informed that all the questionnaires we distributed were anonymous. Participation could be terminated at any time before submitting the completed questionnaire. The study followed the Declaration of Helsinki on Medical Research Involving Human Subjects [32] and the provisions of the Convention for the Protection of Human Rights and Dignity of the Human Being concerning the Application of Biology and Medicine (Oviedo Convention) [33].

10.3 Results

10.3.1 Characteristics of nursing representatives

The participants were nursing assistants and Registered Nurses who were assumed to have palliative care knowledge or experience. Table 10.1 displays descriptive statistics of the demographic variables for our study sample.

There were 104 participants, of which 42.3% ($n = 44$) were male, 49% ($n = 51$) were nursing assistants, and 50% ($n = 53$) were registered nurses. None of these

Tab. 10.1: Descriptive statistics of demographic variables.

Variable	DS	Nursing healthcare professionals (n = 104)			
		Emergency department	Cardiology department	Z, χ^2, or r-value	p
		(n = 79)	(n = 25)		
Gender %(n)	100(104)	100(79)	100(25)	–	–
Female	57.7(60)	46.8(37)	92(23)	15.871[a]	<.001*
Male	42.3(44)	53.2(42)	8(2)		
Age (Y; M ± SD; R)	35.74 ± 11.49; 20–60	35.84 ± 11.90; 20–60	35.44 ± 10.28; 20–59	959.500[b]	.831
Relationship Status %(n)	100(104)	100(79)	100(25)	–	–
Single	24(25)	25.3(20)	20(5)	.052[c]	.820
Married	39.4(41)	38(30)	44(11)		
Divorced	0(0)	0(0)	0(0)		
Cohabitation	36.5(38)	36.7(29)	36(9)		
Widowed	0(0)	0(0)	0(0)		
Education %(n)	100(104)	100(79)	100(25)	–	–
Nursing assistants	49(51)	51.9(41)	40(10)	1.076[a]	.300
Register nurses	51(53)	48.1(38)	60(15)		
TL of WE (Y; M ± SD, R)	13.82 ± 12.41; 1–45	13.59 ± 12.40; 1–39	14.52 ± 12.68; 1–45	935.000[b]	.689

%, percent of participants; *, statistical significance ($p < 0.05$); a, Chi-square test; b, Mann–Whitney U-test; c, Kruskal–Wallis test; DS, descriptive statistics; LT, total length; M, mean; n, sample size; SD, standard deviation; WE, work experience; Y, year.

were widowed or divorced, but 39.4% (n = 41) were married; 36.5% (n=38) were living outside marriage, and 24% (n = 25) were single. In the field of palliative care, 50% (n = 52) had received training; 7.7% (n = 8) had received additional training; and 42.3% (n = 44) had not received any training in palliative care. Respondents were between 20 and 60 years, with mean age of 35.7 years (SD = 11.49). Their working experience ranged from 1 to 45 years, with mean experience of 13.82 years (SD = 12.53). They also differ in years of experience in palliative care, ranging from 0 to 39 years. The average years of experience in palliative care was 2.87 (SD = 7.27).

10.3.2 Knowledge about palliative care

Knowledge of palliative care is important for a patient with heart failure; therefore, we wanted to know the knowledge of nursing healthcare professionals (Tab. 10.2).

Tab. 10.2: Knowledge of the definition and purpose of palliative care.

Palliative care . . .	Emergency department (n = 79)	Cardiology department (n = 25)	Total (n = 104)	p^c
	$\bar{x}^a \pm SD^b$	$\bar{x}^a \pm SD^b$	$\bar{x}^a \pm SD^b$	
. . . a terminally ill patient will be cared for	4.13 ± 1.03	4.40 ± .87	4.19 ± .99	.250
. . . physical symptoms and discomfort, and their relief are the most important	4.29 ± .91	4.56 ± .82	4.36 ± .89	.122
. . . aims to achieve/maintain the best possible quality of life	4.34 ± .89	4.52 ± .82	4.38 ± .87	.328
. . . give psychological support	4.18 ± .90	4.20 ± 1.12	4.18 ± .95	.594
. . . provide spiritual support	4.13 ± .97	4.16 ± 1.14	4.13 ± 1.00	.612
. . . the goal is a dignified death	4.42 ± .84	4.56 ± .82	4.45 ± .84	.378
. . . the extent and intensity of technical and life-sustaining measures should be well considered and discussed with the patient	4.20 ± .79	4.32 ± .90	4.23 ± 82	.364
. . . good communication with and involvement of care partners play an important role	4.38 ± .82	4.56 ± .82	4.42 ± .82	.244

[a]Mean values; [b]standard deviation; [c]Mann–Whitney U-test, *statistical significance ($p < 0.05$).

We found that nursing healthcare professionals in both departments have similar knowledge about the definition and purpose of palliative care. The mean value scores of all statements in ED ranged from 4.13 to 4.42 and from 4.16 to 4.56 points in the cardiology department. We found full and partial agreement in both departments about the knowledge of the definition and purpose of palliative care, and thus no statistically significant differences were observed between the departments.

We also looked at the differences between the general and specialized palliative care between the ED and the cardiology departments (Tab. 10.3).

Table 10.3 shows that 45.2% (n = 47) of participants believe that the differences between general and specialized palliative care are known in the healthcare system; 54.8% (n = 57) do not believe that general and specialized palliative care differences are known. In the emergency room, 45.6% (n=36) also believe this and 54.4% (n = 43) do not believe it. In the cardiology department, 44% (n=11) believe there

Tab. 10.3: Differences between general and specialized palliative care.

Are there differences between general and specialized palliative care in the healthcare system?	Emergency department (n = 79)	Cardiology department (n = 25)	Total (n = 104)
	%(n)	%(n)	%(n)
Yes, the differences between general and specialized palliative care are well known in the healthcare system.	45.6(36)	44(11)	45.2(47)
I do not believe that the differences between general and specialized palliative care are known in the healthcare system.	54.4(43)	56(14)	54.8(57)

n, sample size; %, per cent of participants.

are known differences, and 56% (n=14) believe there are no known differences between general and specialized palliative care in the healthcare system.

10.3.3 Perception of providing palliative care

The differences in the perception of palliative care between the ED and cardiology departments are presented below (Tab. 10.4).

Tab. 10.4: Perception of palliative care.

Palliative care . . .	Emergency department (n = 79)	Cardiology department (n = 25)	Total (n = 104)	p^c
	$\bar{x}^a \pm SD^b$	$\bar{x}^a \pm SD^b$	$\bar{x}^a \pm SD^b$	
. . . the cardiologist, general practitioner, palliative care physician and internist, and nurses should work together (meetings, case conferences, etc.)	4.23 ± 0.91	4.52 ± 0.77	4.30 ± 0.88	0.140
. . . the palliative care provider should only have an advisory role	3.13 ± 1.06	3.36 ± 1.38	3.18 ± 1.39	0.224
. . . clear agreements between all experts/disciplines need to be ensured	4.15 ± 0.80	4.56 ± 0.51	4.25 ± 0.76	0.031[*]
. . . a palliative care doctor must be available for consultation	4.27 ± 0.94	4.68 ± 0.56	4.37 ± 0.88	0.048[*]

Tab. 10.4 (continued)

Palliative care . . .	Emergency department (n = 79)	Cardiology department (n = 25)	Total (n = 104)	p^c
	$\bar{x}^a \pm SD^b$	$\bar{x}^a \pm SD^b$	$\bar{x}^a \pm SD^b$	
. . . a palliative care physician must initiate palliative care	3.65 ± 1.14	3.84 ± 1.34	3.69 ± 1.19	0.301
. . . palliative care must be undertaken by the cardiologist involved	3.42 ± 1.17	3.68 ± 1.38	3.48 ± 1.22	0.224
. . . the general physician present must initiate palliative care	3.75 ± 1.09	3.80 ± 1.32	3.76 ± 1.15	0.553
. . . the internist present must initiate palliative care	3.47 ± 1.20	3.76 ± 1.36	3.54 ± 1.24	0.174
. . . the nurse present must initiate palliative care	3.33 ± 1.23	3.36 ± 1.25	3.34 ± 1.23	0.814
. . . continuing training should be available to all practitioners	4.24 ± 0.90	4.68 ± 0.56	4.35 ± 0.85	0.033*
. . . collective transdisciplinary training should be offered to all physicians involved in a patient's care	4.10 ± 0.99	4.72 ± 0.54	4.25 ± 0.94	0.004*
. . . palliative care should be set up in an institution (hospital/nursing home)	4.16 ± 0.98	4.44 ± 0.92	4.23 ± 0.97	0.158
. . . a palliative care physician should mostly provide treatments	3.72 ± 0.97	4.08 ± 0.99	3.81 ± 0.99	0.098
. . . a cardiologist should mostly carry out treatments	3.28 ± 1.12	3.28 ± 1.31	3.28 ± 1.16	0.969
. . . a general practitioner should carry out most treatments	3.34 ± 1.14	3.60 ± 1.23	3.40 ± 1.16	0.353
. . . an internist should carry out most treatments	3.23 ± 1.07	3.40 ± 1.23	3.27 ± 1.11	0.673
. . . a nurse should carry out most treatments	3.54 ± 1.04	3.24 ± 1.09	3.47 ± 1.05	0.172

[a]Mean values; [b]standard deviation; [c]Mann–Whitney U-test, *statistical significance ($p < 0.05$).

The data show a statistically significant difference between the ED and cardiology departments regarding the perception of implementing palliative care. Differences emerged in the statements about clear information flow ($p = 0.031$; $\bar{x}_{ED} = 4.15 \pm 0.80$; $\bar{x}_{cardiology} = 4.56 \pm 0.51$), training in palliative care ($p = 0.033$; $\bar{x}_{ED} = 4.27 \pm 0.94$; $\bar{x}_{cardiology} = 4.68 \pm 0.56$), and ensuring consultation and support from the transdisciplinary palliative care team ($p = 0.048$; $\bar{x}_{ED} = 4.27 \pm 0.94$; $\bar{x}_{cardiology} = 4.68 \pm 0.56$). Moreover, further education should be available to all nursing healthcare professionals and they should be offered collective training in palliative care, including the physicians involved in the patient's care ($p = 0.004$; $\bar{x}_{ED} = 4.10 \pm 0.99$; $\bar{x}_{cardiology} = 4.72 \pm 0.54$).

10.3.4 Attitudes towards palliative care

Below are the results about differences in attitudes towards palliative care in patients with heart failure between the ED and the cardiology departments (Tab. 10.5).

Tab. 10.5: Attitudes towards palliative care.

Items	Emergency department ($n = 79$)	Cardiology department ($n = 25$)	Total ($n = 104$)	p^c
	$\bar{x}^a \pm SD^b$	$\bar{x}^a \pm SD^b$	$\bar{x}^a \pm SD^b$	
There is a need for palliative care in treating patients with heart failure.	3.72 ± 0.91	4.28 ± 0.94	3.86 ± 0.94	0.003[*]
Demand for palliative care in treating patients with heart failure is increasing.	3.46 ± 0.86	3.96 ± 1.06	3.58 ± 0.93	0.009[*]
De-escalation of therapy makes more sense than continuing current treatment.	3.30 ± 0.82	3.84 ± 0.75	3.43 ± 0.84	0.004[*]
Cardiology, general medicine, and internal medicine can learn from expertise in palliative care.	3.63 ± 0.82	3.96 ± 0.79	3.71 ± 0.82	0.062
More intensive care is possible through palliative care.	3.70 ± 0.87	4 ± 0.87	3.77 ± 0.78	0.087
The quality of life of patients with advanced heart failure will be further reduced by introducing invasive therapies such as cardiac assist devices.	3.63 ± 0.88	3.88 ± 0.78	3.69 ± 0.86	0.193
The quality of remaining life can be improved in palliative care.	4.11 ± 0.85	4.44 ± 0.58	4.19 ± 0.80	0.112
Patients do not require palliative care.	3.06 ± 1.04	3.24 ± 1.33	3.11 ± 1.11	0.372
It is difficult to determine the right time to start palliative care because of the difficulty in assessing disease progression.	3.63 ± 0.88	3.76 ± 0.97	3.66 ± 0.60	0.524

Tab. 10.5 (continued)

Items	Emergency department (n = 79)	Cardiology department (n = 25)	Total (n = 104)	p^c
	$\bar{x}^a \pm SD^b$	$\bar{x}^a \pm SD^b$	$\bar{x}^a \pm SD^b$	
Complex heart failure therapies can also be used in very elderly patients. Therefore, palliative care is not necessary.	2.99 ± 1.08	2.84 ± 1.21	2.95 ± 1.11	0.662
Major advances have been made in the treatment of heart failure. Therefore, palliative care is not necessary.	2.92 ± 0.92	3.16 ± 1.21	2.98 ± 0.99	0.313
Palliative care can be taken over entirely by the attending general practitioner/cardiologist/internist.	3.29 ± 1.06	3.60 ± 1.12	3.37 ± 1.08	0.220
A patient with chronic heart failure does not feel he/she is in a situation for palliative care.	3.43 ± 0.84	3.48 ± 0.92	3.44 ± 0.86	0.761
Patients may refuse further escalation of treatment when palliative care is available.	3.41 ± 0.81	3.92 ± 1.04	3.53 ± 0.89	0.005*

[a]Mean values; [b]standard deviation; [c]Mann–Whitney U-test; *statistical significance ($p < 0.05$).

Regarding nursing healthcare professionals' attitudes towards palliative care for patients with heart failure, there were statistically significant differences between the ED and the cardiology departments in some of the statements, namely that there remains a need for palliative care in treating patients with heart failure ($p = 0.003$; $\bar{x}_{ED} = 3.72 \pm 0.91$; $\bar{x}_{cardiology} = 4.28 \pm .94$). There is an increasing demand for palliative care in treating patients with heart failure ($p = 0.009$; $\bar{x}_{ED} = 3.46 \pm 0.86$; $\bar{x}_{cardiology} = 3.96 \pm 0.79$). Opinions also differed on de-escalation of therapy, which makes more sense than a continuation ($p = 0.004$; $\bar{x}_{ED} = 3.30 \pm 0.82$; $\bar{x}_{cardiology} = 3.84 \pm 0.75$), and on the idea that patients should be able to refuse further escalation of treatment when palliative care is available ($p = 0.005$; $\bar{x}_{ED} = 3.41 \pm 0.81$; $\bar{x}_{cardiology} = 3.92 \pm 1.04$).

We also looked at whether there were differences in the thresholds of palliative care benefits between the ED and cardiology departments (Tab. 10.6).

When comparing the ED and cardiology departments about the usefulness of palliative care for patients with chronic heart failure, 64.6% ($n = 51$) of the participants in the ED consider palliative care useful to patients. Only 10.1% ($n = 8$) consider it not useful, and 25.3% ($n = 20$) are unable to make up their minds. In the cardiology department, 84% ($n = 21$) felt that palliative care was useful, 8% ($n = 2$) could not decide, and 8% ($n = 2$) felt that palliative care was not useful. Overall, 69.2% ($n = 72$) agree that palliative care is useful, 9.6% ($n = 10$) disagree, and 21.2% ($n = 22$) could not decide.

Tab. 10.6: The benefits of palliative care.

Is palliative care beneficial for patients with chronic heart failure?	Emergency department (n = 79)	Cardiology department (n = 25)	Total (n = 104)
	%(n)	%(n)	%(n)
Yes, I think palliative care for patients with chronic heart failure is beneficial.	64.6(51)	84(21)	69.2(72)
I do not think palliative care for patients with chronic heart failure is beneficial.	10.1(8)	8(2)	9.6(10)
I have no opinion on this issue.	25.3(20)	8(2)	21.2(22)

n, sample size; %, per cent of participants.

Table 10.7 displays a correlation between work experience and nursing healthcare professionals' attitudes towards palliative care for heart failure patients.

Table 10.7 shows the correlation matrix of work experience and nursing healthcare professionals' attitudes towards palliative care. A significant positive association exists between the sub-domains related to attitudes towards palliative care and work experience. The correlation coefficient itself ranged between 0.001 and 1. The range for strong correlation was between 0.75 and 0.84. Of these, work experience and D13 ("A patient with chronic heart failure does not feel that he or she is in a situation for palliative care") ($r_s = 0.84$; $n = 104$; $p < 0.001$) was the strongest. The range for moderate correlation was between 0.46 and 0.59. Of the range of correlation coefficients, the highest coefficient was between work experience and D8 ("Patients do not require palliative care") ($r_s = 0.59$; $n = 104$; $p < 0.001$). The range for weakest correlation was between 0.12 and 0.33. Of this, the highest correlation coefficient was between work experience and D14 ("Patients may refuse further escalation of treatment when palliative care is available") ($r_s = 0.33$; $n = 104$; $p < 0.001$). The range for negligible correlation was between 0.001 and 0.04. Of these, work experience correlates most strongly with D4 ("Cardiology, general medicine and internal medicine can learn from expertise in palliative care") ($r_s = 0.04$; $n = 104$; $p = 0.038$).

10.4 Discussion

This study investigated nursing healthcare professionals' knowledge, perceptions, and attitudes towards palliative care in patients with heart failure in the ED and cardiology departments. Nursing healthcare professionals in both departments had similar views on their palliative care knowledge, with scores ranging from 4.13 to 4.42 in the ED and from 4.16 to 4.56 in the cardiology departments. In the context of

Tab. 10.7: Spearman correlations matrix of work experience and nursing healthcare professionals' attitudes towards palliative care.

	TL of WE	D1	D2	D3	D4	D5	D6	D7	D8	D9	D10	D11	D12	D13	D14
TL of WE	1	0.12	0.47	0.75	0.04*	0.47	0.32	0.12	0.59	0.24	0.53	0.51	0.46	0.84	0.33
D1	0.12	1	0.001*	0.01*	0.001*	0.001*	0.001*	0.001*	0.48	0.06	0.47	0.45	0.31	0.19	0.20
D2	0.47	0.001*	1	0.001*	0.001*	0.001*	0.001*	0.01*	0.66	0.34	0.51	0.13	0.001*	0.001*	0.02*
D3	0.75	0.01*	0.001*	1	0.001*	0.01	0.001*	0.07	0.04*	0.05*	0.02*	0.001*	0.001*	0.42	0.001*
D4	0.04*	0.001*	0.001*	0.001*	1	0.001*	0.001*	0.001*	0.10	0.001*	0.48	0.01*	0.03*	0.25	0.08
D5	0.47	0.001*	0.001*	0.01*	0.001*	1	0.001*	0.01*	0.45	0.05*	0.60	0.16	0.94	0.01*	0.27
D6	0.32	0.001*	0.001*	0.001*	0.001*	0.001*	1	0.01*	0.09	0.04*	0.24	0.001*	0.06	0.001*	0.13
D7	0.12	0.001*	0.01*	0.07	0.001*	0.001*	0.01*	1	0.92	0.02*	0.82	0.75	0.79	0.24	0.15
D8	0.59	0.48	0.66	0.04*	0.10	0.45	0.09	0.92	1	0.001*	0.001*	0.001*	0.29	0.01*	0.02*
D9	0.24	0.06	0.34	0.05*	0.001*	0.05*	0.04*	0.02*	0.001*	1	0.001*	0.001*	0.04*	0.01*	0.01*
D10	0.53	0.47	0.51	0.02*	0.48	0.60	0.24	0.82	0.001*	0.001*	1	0.001*	0.02*	0.07	0.03*
D11	0.51	0.45	0.13	0.001*	0.01*	0.16	0.001*	0.75	0.001*	0.001*	0.001*	1	0.001*	0.01*	0.001*
D12	0.46	0.31	0.001*	0.001*	0.03*	0.94	0.06	0.79	0.29	0.04*	0.02*	0.001*	1	0.001*	0.001*
D13	0.84	0.19	0.001*	0.42	0.25	0.01*	0.001*	0.24	0.01*	0.01*	0.07	0.01*	0.001*	1	0.001*
D14	0.33	0.20	0.02*	0.001*	0.08	0.27	0.13	0.15	0.02*	0.01*	0.03*	0.001*	0.001*	0.001*	1

D1, there is a need for palliative care in the treatment of patients with heart failure; D2, demand for palliative care in the treatment of patients with heart failure is increasing; D3, de-escalation of therapy makes more sense than continuing current therapy; D4, cardiology, general medicine, and internal medicine can learn from expertise in palliative care; D5, more intensive care is possible through palliative care; D6, the quality of life of patients with advanced heart failure will be further reduced by the introduction of invasive therapies such as heart-assist devices; D7, quality of remaining life can be improved with palliative care; D8, patients do not require palliative care; D9, it is difficult to determine the right time to start palliative care because of the difficulty in assessing disease progression; D10, complex heart failure therapies can also be used in very elderly patients; palliative care is therefore not necessary; D11, major advances have been made in the treatment of heart failure. Palliative care is therefore not necessary; D12, palliative care can be taken over entirely by the attending general practitioner/cardiologist/internist; D13, a patient with chronic heart failure does not feel that he/she are in a situation for palliative care; D14, patients may refuse further escalation of treatment when palliative care is available; TL of WE, total length of work experience; *statistical significance (p < 0.05).

barriers to palliative care, we found that both departments agree, with the mean value ranging from 3.01 to 3.92. However, according to the mean value of the statements, the biggest barrier is that the care partners want everything possible to cure the patient, which is what health professionals in the ED and cardiology departments consider the biggest barrier.

Nursing healthcare professionals in the cardiology departments have the same knowledge with regard to the definition and purpose of palliative care as those in the ED. The biggest difference was that cardiology departments were more likely to agree that physical symptoms, discomfort, and relief were most important, and that the terminal patient would be cared for in palliative care. Alshammari et al. [34] also came to similar conclusions, adding that they are united in their knowledge of pain management and distress symptom management.

From our survey, both departments placed the dignified death of patients first, followed closely by the important role of good communication with and the involvement of care partners in palliative care. Ziehm et al. [16] stress the importance of fostering good communication between the healthcare professionals, patients, and care partners, and the need for overcoming such perceived barriers. The third most important purpose of palliative care is defined as the aim to achieve/preserve the best possible quality of life for patients. Both departments define the third most important purpose of palliative care as, preserving the quality of life for patients. Many studies [35–38] have also found that early integration of palliative care in the acute treatment of a patient with a chronic non-communicable disease is a key component in maintaining the quality of life and preserving their dignity. Nursing healthcare professionals were presented with different views on palliative care, to which they responded with the extent to which they agreed with these views. We found a statistically significant association between work experience and the item "Cardiology, general medicine, and internal medicine can learn from the expertise in palliative care" ($r_s = 0.04$; $n = 104$; $p = 0.038$). In the study by Ziehm et al. [16], health professionals in both departments overwhelmingly agreed with the view that cardiology, general medicine, and internal medicine can learn from expertise in palliative care. This was the view most strongly shared by 90.9% of all nursing healthcare professionals. Our survey found that the mean value for this question was 3.71, indicating that health professionals are more likely to agree than disagree.

Despite advances in the recognition and treatment, heart failure is not yet eradicated and remains one of the most common reasons for patient hospitalization [39]. Palliative care provides a mechanism whereby the patient's quality of care during the end of life period can be maintained. Nursing healthcare professionals should be aware of the importance and benefits of palliative care for patients with heart failure, and efforts should be made to include such patients in palliative care. There is a need to enhance education on palliative care, improve management of heart failure, and foster open communication within and across transdisciplinary healthcare teams on treatment strategies. It is important to start early by talking to the patient about their prognosis. However, this requires a person-centred planning [40, 41].

This study has several limitations that need to be considered. For this study, we used a convenience sample of nursing healthcare professionals. The results should not be generalized and we should be cautious in applying our findings, as the survey sample was realistically small and local. The cross-sectional design limits conclusions about causality, as it only describes variables that influence or interact with each other. Self-assessment of nursing healthcare professionals' knowledge, perceptions, and attitudes was based on subjective judgements rather than objective criteria.

The findings are not representative of the entire population of nursing healthcare professionals in Slovenia or worldwide, but specifically about nursing healthcare professionals in the ED and cardiology departments. To explore the attitudes of nursing healthcare professionals towards palliative care for patients with heart failure further, it may be useful to adopt a qualitative design to gain a broader understanding of the experiences of nursing healthcare professionals and to identify some of the dimensions that the survey was not able to perceive. A qualitative approach could also provide insights into developing new factors to improve palliative care in patients with heart failure.

10.5 Conclusions

We found no differences in palliative care knowledge of nursing healthcare professionals between the cardiology and ED departments. Nursing healthcare professionals in the cardiology departments have the same knowledge of the definition and purpose of palliative care as those in the ED. Half of the nursing healthcare professionals cannot decide whether they are satisfied or not with their knowledge of palliative care. Still, the survey shows that more of them are satisfied than dissatisfied. We recommend organizing additional and continuous training on palliative care, as almost half of the nursing healthcare professionals who took part in our survey had not received any training in palliative care.

References

[1] Hart PL, Spiva L, Kimble LP. Nurses' knowledge of heart failure education principles survey: A psychometric study. J Clin Nurs, 2011, 20(21–22), 3020–3028.
[2] Ambrosy AP, Fonarow GC, Butler J, Chioncel O, Greene SJ, Vaduganathan M, et al. The global health and economic burden of hospitalisations for heart failure: Lessons learned from hospitalised heart failure registries. J Am Coll Cardiol, 2014, 63(12), 1123–1133.

[3]   Maggioni AP, Dahlström U, Filippatos G, Chioncel O, Crespo Leiro M, Drozdz J, et al. EURObservational research programme: Regional differences and 1-year follow-up results of the heart failure pilot survey (ESC-HF Pilot). Eur J Heart Fail, 2013, 15(7), 808–817.

[4]   Voga G, Vrtovec B. Srčno popuščanje. In: Košnik M, Mrevlje F, Štajer D, Černelč P, Koželj M, Andoljšek D, et al., eds. Interna medicina. 4th ed. Ljubljana, Littera picta, 2011.

[5]   Claret PG, Stiell IG, Yan JW, Clement CM, Rowe BH, Calder LA, et al. Characteristics and outcomes for acute heart failure in elderly patients presenting to the ED. Am J Emerg Med, 2016, 34(11), 2159–2166.

[6]   Bloom MW, Greenberg B, Jaarsma T, Januzzi JL, Lam CSP, Maggioni AP, et al. Heart failure with reduced ejection fraction. Nat Rev Dis Primers, 2017, 3(1), 17058.

[7]   Boisvert S, Proulx-Belhumeur A, Gonçalves N, Doré M, Francoeur J, Gallani MC. An integrative literature review on nursing interventions aimed at increasing self-care among heart failure patients. Rev Lat Am Enfermagem, 2015, 23(4), 753–768.

[8]   Fernandes Pedro J, Reis-Pina P. Palliative care in patients with advanced heart failure: A systematic review. Acta Médica Portuguesa, 2022, 35(2), 111.

[9]   Mierendorf S. Palliative care in the emergency department. Perm J, 2014, 18(2), 77–85.

[10] Bogataj A, Cerar A. Akutno srčno popuščanje – obravnava v urgentnem centru. In: Prosen G, ed. Šola urgence 2018: Zbornik VI Šola urgence, 2018, 1 letnik, 2 cikel; Kardiologija, pulmologija in vaskularna medicina, Laško, 30 november in 1 december 2018. Ljubljana, Slovensko združenje za urgentno medicino, 2018.

[11] Pang PS, Collins SP, Ò M, Bueno H, Diercks DB, Di Somma S, et al. Editor's choice-the role of the emergency department in the management of acute heart failure: An international perspective on education and research. Eur Heart J Acute Cardiovasc Care, 2017, 6(5), 421–429.

[12] Lipinski M, Eagles D, Fischer LM, Mielniczuk L, Stiell IG. Heart failure and palliative care in the emergency department. Emerg Med J, 2018, 35(12), 726–729.

[13] Ò M, Peacock FW, McMurray JJ, Bueno H, Christ M, Maisel AS, et al. European society of cardiology – acute cardiovascular care association position paper on safe discharge of acute heart failure patients from the emergency department. Eur Heart J Acute Cardiovasc Care, 2017, 6(4), 311–320.

[14] Schnell-Hoehn K, Estrella-Holder E, Avery L. N028 cardiac nurses' knowledge of palliative care at a tertiary care facility. Can J Cardiol, 2012, 28(5), S428–S9.

[15] Grudzen CR, Richardson LD, Morrison M, Cho E, Sean Morrison R. Palliative care needs of seriously Ill, older adults presenting to the emergency department. Acad Emergency Med, 2010, 17(11), 1253–1257.

[16] Ziehm J, Farin E, Schäfer J, Woitha K, Becker G, Köberich S. Palliative care for patients with heart failure: Facilitators and barriers – a cross sectional survey of German health care professionals. BMC Health Serv Res, 2016, 16(a), 361.

[17] Delgado JM, Ruppar TM. Health literacy in older latinos with heart failure: A systematic review. J Cardiovasc Nurs, 2017, 32(2), 125–134.

[18] Sanad HM. Nurses' knowledge and attitude towards management of patients with heart failure. J Adv Pharm Educ Res, 2017, 7(7), 387–393.

[19] Ieraci S. Palliative care in the emergency department. Emergency Med Australas, 2013, 25, 112–113.

[20] Jelinek GA, Marck CH, Weiland TJ, Philip J, Boughey M, Weil J, et al. Caught in the middle: Tensions around the emergency department care of people with advanced cancer. Emerg Med Australas, 2013, 25(2), 154–160.

[21] Meo N, Hwang U, Morrison RS. Resident perceptions of palliative care training in the emergency department. J Palliat Med, 2011, 14(5), 548–555.

[22] Smith AK, Fisher J, Schonberg MA, Pallin DJ, Block SD, Forrow L, et al. Am I doing the right thing? Provider perspectives on improving palliative care in the emergency department. Ann Emerg Med, 2009, 54(1), 86–93, .e1.

[23] Stone SC, Mohanty S, Grudzen CR, Shoenberger J, Asch S, Kubricek K, et al. Emergency medicine physicians' perspectives of providing palliative care in an emergency department. J Palliat Med, 2011, 14(12), 1333–1338.

[24] Todd KH. Practically speaking: Emergency medicine and the palliative care movement. Emerg Med Australas, 2012, 24(1), 4–6.

[25] Lukin W, Douglas C, O'Connor A. Palliative care in the emergency department: An oxymoron or just good medicine? Emerg Med Australas, 2012, 24(1), 102–104.

[26] McIlvennan CK, Allen LA. Palliative care in patients with heart failure. Bmj, 2016, 353, i1010.

[27] Lowey SE. Palliative care in the management of patients with advanced heart failure. In: Islam MS, ed. Heart failure: From research to clinical practice: Volume 3. Cham, Springer International Publishing, 2018, 295–311.

[28] Polit DF, Beck CT. Nursing research: Generating and assessing evidence for nursing practice. 11th ed. Philadelphia, Wolters Kluwer.

[29] von Elm E, Altman DG, Egger M, Pocock SJ, Gøtzsche PC, Vandenbroucke JP. The strengthening the reporting of observational studies in epidemiology (STROBE) statement: Guidelines for reporting observational studies. PLoS Med, 2007, 4(10), e296.

[30] Cochran WG. Sampling techniques. 3rd ed. New York, John Wiley & Sons, 1977.

[31] Schober P, Boer C, Schwarte LA. Correlation coefficients: Appropriate use and interpretation. Anesth Analg, 2018, 126(5), 1763–1768.

[32] Council of Europe. Convention for the protection of human rights and dignity of the human being with regard to the application of biology and medicine (European tratyseries-no. 164). Oviedo, Council of Europe.

[33] World Medical Association. Declaration of Helsinki. Ethical principles for medical research involving human subjects. Jahrbuch Für Wissenschaft und Ethik, 2009, 14(1), 233–238.

[34] Alshammari F, Sim J, Lapkin S, Stephens M. Registered nurses' knowledge, attitudes and beliefs about end-of-life care in non-specialist palliative care settings: A mixed studies review. Nurse Educ Pract, 2022, 59, 103294.

[35] Ahluwalia SC, Chen C, Raaen L, Motala A, Walling AM, Chamberlin M, et al. A systematic review in support of the national consensus project clinical practice guidelines for quality palliative care, Fourth Edition. J Pain Symptom Manage, 2018, 56(6), 831–870.

[36] Amador S, Sampson EL, Goodman C, Robinson L. A systematic review and critical appraisal of quality indicators to assess optimal palliative care for older people with dementia. Palliat Med, 2019, 33(4), 415–429.

[37] Bausewein C, Simon ST, Pralong A, Radbruch L, Nauck F, Voltz R. Palliative care of adult patients with cancer. Dtsch Arztebl Int, 2015, 112(50), 863–870.

[38] Durepos P, Wickson-Griffiths A, Hazzan AA, Kaasalainen S, Vastis V, Battistella L, et al. Assessing palliative care content in dementia care guidelines: A systematic review. J Pain Symptom Manage, 2017, 53(4), 804–813.

[39] Adler ED, Bui QM. Performing sit down medicine in a stand-up place: Is it time for palliative care in the emergency department? Emergency Med J, 2018, 35(12), 730.

[40] Kmetec S, Fekonja Z, Kolarič JČ, Reljić NM, McCormack B, Sigurðardóttir ÁK, et al. Components for providing person-centred palliative healthcare: An umbrella review. Int J Nurs Stud, 2022, 125, 104111.

[41] Uppal S. The challenge of palliative care in heart failure. Br J Cardiac Nurs, 2013, 8(2), 90–95.

Nataša Mlinar Reljić, Fiona Timmins, Zvonka Fekonja,
Sergej Kmetec, Blanka Kores Plesničar, Majda Pajnkihar,
Tatjana Ribič

11 The role and meaning of spirituality in older people living with dementia: a systematic review of qualitative studies

Abstract

Background: Spiritual care can improve the cognitive ability and the associated activities, and help raise self-esteem and self-sufficiency in older people with dementia. It creates hope, helps find purpose and inner peace, and improve their sense of satisfaction with life. Thus, spirituality is a crucial element in providing nursing care for older people. This chapter aims to present the role and meaning of spirituality for people with dementia.

Methods: Systematic review of qualitative studies was performed. CINAHL, PubMed, Science Direct, EBSCO host databases, and reference lists were searched for studies published until April 2021. The Qualitative Assessment and Review Instrument was used to assess the quality of studies. Data was synthesized using thematic analysis.

Results: Ten studies were included. Two main themes: (1) spirituality as an inner source of power; and (2) spirituality as connectedness, described the role and meaning of spirituality.

Discussion: Spirituality is an inner source that gives people with dementia the strength to face dementia. It highlights the role and meaning of connectedness with the self and with others. Relationships with family and the community are essential reflections of spiritual life, and represent a source of incentive and joy for older people with dementia.

Keywords: spirituality, older people, dementia, systematic review

11.1 Introduction

It is well understood internationally that people live longer, with an increasing incidence of multi-morbidity and an increased likelihood of using hospital and healthcare services. The increased risk of dementia is an additional burden associated with longevity that can profoundly impact a person's quality of life and increase the likelihood of engaging with the healthcare system and being dependent on its support [1, 2]. Physical care needs are prioritized in hospitals, residential, and community settings [3]. However, this care creates gaps in the care of older people with dementia as they may have profound psychosocial and spiritual needs due to their cognitive decline.

People with dementia require a person-centred and relationship-orientated humane approach, and an environment that helps them connect to their personhood [4, 5]. There are increasing calls for a reorientation of the care for people with dementia, which should focus on the fundamental aspects of care delivery, especially relationships and providing respectful, humane care [6]. Understanding spirituality is one such issue. Although conflated with religion, it is quite a distinct area that describes a person's search for meaning in life, their sense of connectedness, and the experience of transcendence [7]. There is no consistent definition of spirituality in literature, but definitions go beyond religious and cultural definitions [8]. Spirituality is often associated with an individual's relationship with the world and their personal beliefs [9], their individual and subjective experience of themselves and with the dimensions outside, and of the connection with nature and higher powers [7]. Spirituality is described as a universal, very personal, and individual experience that captures each person's exclusive ability, as the core and essence of being a person, which permeates the entire structure of a person and a being worthy of dignity and respect [8].

Expressing spiritual needs depends on cultural beliefs and practices, and personal beliefs and practices. However, spirituality does not extinguish dementia [10]. For people with dementia, dissatisfaction due to physical discomfort, emotional distress, and social isolation may be reflected in the way they express their different spiritual needs [8]. Further, physical and mental changes associated with dementia can be perceived as the loss of personhood and oneself [11]. The effects of stressful events in life can be indirectly reduced by satisfying their spiritual needs, including the fear of the unknown, even death, and help achieve transcendence and contribute to their spiritual development [12]. Spirituality enables an individual to find hope, meaning, and purpose in life and inner peace; it improves one's sense of satisfaction with life, helps them cope with suffering and loss, and connects to one's personhood [13]. Therefore, providing spiritual care is crucial in helping people cope with their dementia condition [14], which is why the spiritual aspects of nursing are valued in practice. As such, spiritual support for older people is gaining attention in the published literature [12].

Previous reviews about spirituality in people with dementia have focused on the different aspects of spirituality. Spirituality as a way of dealing with the early stages of Alzheimer's dementia was explored [15], and its features and its impact on people with late-stage dementia was examined [16]. Furthermore, how spirituality influenced people diagnosed with dementia [14] was researched and the spiritual experiences of people with dementia was explored from a qualitative perspective [13]. However, no review has specifically examined the role and meaning of spirituality in people with dementia to date. The chapter aimed to find meaning and interpret the role of the spirituality on older people with dementia.

11.2 Methods

A systematic review, followed by a thematic synthesis of qualitative research [17], was carried out. Meta-synthesis is the interpretative integration of findings from qualitative studies and allows a new interpretation of the research phenomenon [18]. The Preferred Reporting Items for Systematic Reviews and Meta-Analyses (PRISMA) guidelines were followed for reporting [19].

11.2.1 Search strategy

The PEO approach guidelines were used to create the research question [20]. The research question of this systematic review was: What is the meaning and role (O) of Spirituality (E) in people with dementia (P)? The inclusion and exclusion criteria for the review are outlined in Tab. 11.1.

Tab. 11.1: Inclusion and exclusion criteria relating to the PEO research question.

PEO parameters	Inclusion criteria	Exclusion criteria
Population	Older people Diagnosis of dementia	Young adults People not diagnosed with dementia Nurses, family caregivers
Exposure	Spirituality	Non-spirituality
Outcome	Meaning Role	Research does not include meaning and role
Study type	Qualitative methodology design	Quantitative methodology design, mixed methods, case studies Reviews, meta-synthesis, meta-analysis, Editor letters, commentaries

The search was conducted using search terms in the English language: dementia, older adults, spiritual, meaning, and role, with their synonyms and Boolean operators. The final search was run as: ((demen* OR Alzheim*) AND (elderly OR "older adults" OR "older people") AND ("spiritual care" OR spirit*) AND role AND meaning*). The MeSH terms search was also used. We determined the articles published in English between 1990 and April 2021 in the following databases: CINAHL, PubMed, Science Direct, EBSCO host. After the key articles were identified, additional searches were carried out using the "Related Articles" search feature in the PubMed database. Reference lists of included studies were also searched.

11.2.2 Selection process

The identified records were screened in three steps. First, the identified papers were imported into the Mendeley program. After duplicates were removed, the two authors independently evaluated the titles and abstracts against the inclusion and exclusion criteria, and those not meeting the inclusion criteria were excluded. We used the Qualitative Assessment and Review Instrument (QARI) to assess the quality of these papers. The QARI quality assessment checklist consisted of 10-items to determine the extent to which a qualitative study addressed the possibility of bias in its research design, conduct, and analysis [21]. All studies meeting the inclusion criteria were independently assessed for methodological quality by the two researchers, and the co-authors arbitrated disagreements between them.

11.2.3 Data extraction and synthesis

Data extraction was based on the aim to find a deeper meaning and interpret the role of the spirituality of people living with dementia. The extracted data's headings were the following: the place where the study was conducted, sampling, methodology with research design, and the outcome themes. Data was extracted by three researchers and subsequently checked by the lead author. The thematic approach [17] was adopted to analyse and synthesize the data in three steps: (1) Line-by-line coding to identify free codes; (2) organizing free codes into descriptive primary and secondary level subthemes; and (3) developing main themes. Discussions involving all the authors were conducted to reach a consensus on naming the two main themes.

11.3 Results

During the initial search, 1,654 records were identified. After removing duplicates, 1,633 articles were screened for relevance, by title and abstract, and removed those ($n = 1,580$) that did not meet the inclusion criteria. Fifty-three complete articles were evaluated for eligibility, and 43 articles were excluded as they did not focus on dementia, spirituality, and older people. One study [22] also included relatives, which we nevertheless included in the analysis, as the data analysis in the article was given separately for relatives and for people living with dementia. In this manner, ten articles were included in the critical appraisal (Fig. 11.1).

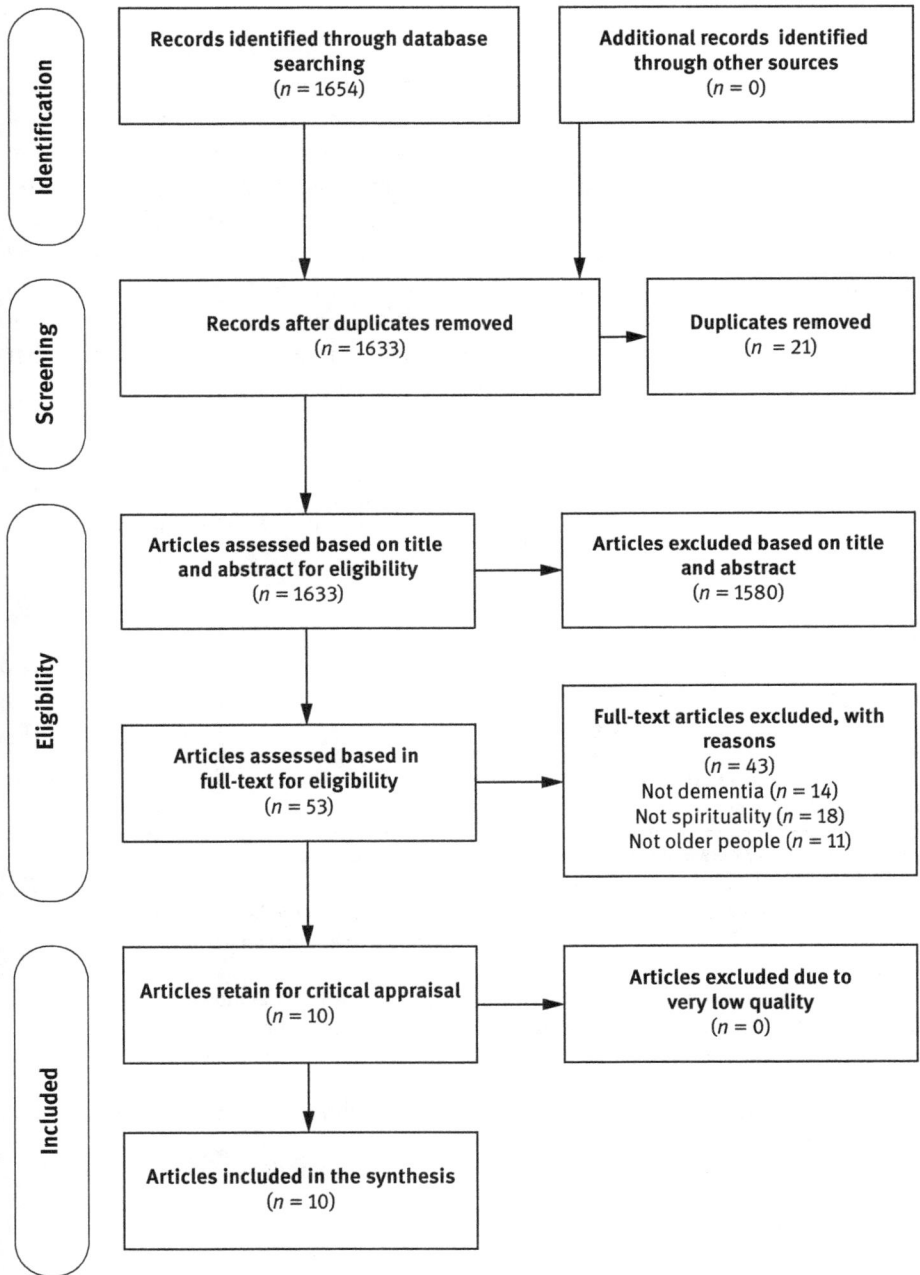

Fig. 11.1: The flow chart illustrates the search process [19].

11.3.1 Study quality appraisal

The selected studies met the primary considerations relevant to our research. The studies' most common weakness was in the statement –the researcher's theoretical or cultural orientation. Only one study [11] clearly stated the researcher's cultural orientation. Also, there was an evident lack of information regarding how the researcher influenced the study. The relationship between the participants and the researcher was clearly stated only in two studies [11, 23]. Further, the studies lacked information on reporting the congruity between the philosophical and research methodologies, as presented in Tab. 11.2. However, in keeping with guidance on these criteria and agreement within the research team, all ten studies broadly met the criteria and were retained for closer examination.

Tab. 11.2: Critical appraisal of included studies.

Study/criteria	1	2	3	4	5	6	7	8	9	10	Overall appraisal
Beuscher and Grando [15]	+	+	+	+	+	−	−	+	+	+	8/10
Dalby et al. [11]	+	+	+	+	+	+	+	+	?	+	9/10
Gardiner [24]	+	+	+	+	+	−	−	+	+	+	8/10
MacKinlay [25]	+	+	+	+	+	−	−	+	+	+	8/10
McGee and Myers [26]	−	+	+	+	+	−	−	+	+	+	7/10
Phinney [27]	+	+	+	+	+	−	−	+	+	+	8/10
Snyder [28]	+	+	+	+	+	−	−	+	?	+	7/10
Sullivan and Beard [22]	+	+	+	+	+	−	−	+	+	+	8/10
Trevitt and MacKinlay [23]	+	+	+	+	+	−	+	+	+	+	9/10
Trevitt and MacKinlay [29]	+	+	+	+	+	−	−	+	+	+	8/10

1: Is there congruity between the stated philosophical perspective and the research methodology?
2: Is there congruity between the research methodology and the research question or objectives?
3: Is there congruity between the research methodology and the methods used to collect data?
4: Is there congruity between the research methodology, and the representation and analysis of data?
5: Is there congruity between the research methodology and the interpretation of the results?
6: Is there a statement locating the researcher, culturally or theoretically?
7: Is the influence of the researcher on the research, and vice-versa, addressed?
8: Are the participants and their voices adequately represented?
9: Is the research ethical, according to the current criteria or for recent studies, and is there evidence of ethical approval by an appropriate body?
10: Do the conclusions drawn in the research report, flow from the analysis or interpretation of the data?
+, yes; −, no; ?, unclear.

11.3.2 Study characteristics

All studies used a qualitative research design – ethnographic approach [15], phenomenology [11, 24, 27], grounded theory [25], and observation [15, 27, 29]. Interview, as a data collecting method, was used the most frequently [11, 15, 22, 23, 25–29]. Also, focus groups were used for collecting data [22]. Six studies were conducted in the United States, three in Australia, and one in Europe. The total sample from all the included studies presents 177 older people with dementia. Detailed descriptions are provided in Tab. 11.3.

11.3.3 Understanding spirituality and meaning in older people living with dementia

Line-by-line coding of all the studies resulted in the identification of free codes (*n* = 86). Based on that the free codes, we developed primary subthemes (*n* = 13), secondary subthemes (*n* = 4) and two main themes: (1) spirituality as an inner source of power and (2) spirituality as connectedness (Tab. 11.4).

Spirituality as an inner source of power

First main them, *Spirituality as an inner source of power*, was developed from two secondary subthemes: (1) facing dementia and (2) facing oneself.

Facing dementia: Having to face dementia is often accompanied by bouts of anger and the feeling that they have somehow been wronged [28]. However, some authors report that people with dementia see their situation as an opportunity to mature and grow, and think that the disease may enable their souls to develop spiritually [11, 24]. Many studies we analysed [11, 23, 25, 27, 28] show that people with dementia often ask questions that mostly remain unanswered. The question "why" is widespread: "why me, can I manage, why did I become ill [11], why exactly me [28]?" Such questions often remain without answers or satisfying answers, bringing unrest, frustration, and uncertainty to older people with dementia [13]. Due to their awareness of mortality, such individuals can become even more vulnerable [25].

In facing dementia, hope is one of the essential inner sources of power and reflects the spiritual maturity of older people with dementia, according to numerous studies [11, 15, 22, 28]. Hope is the inner power that gives strength to the older person with dementia to cope with such a severe illness and the resulting situation [28]. At the same time, it helps an older person to accept the disease and recognize new opportunities for which many are also grateful [22, 28]. Hope is the expression

Tab. 11.3: Overview of the included studies.

References, country	Objective	Sample	Methodology	Identified themes
Beuscher and Grando [15], USA	Describes how individuals with early stages of Alzheimer's dementia use spirituality to cope with the losses of self-esteem, independence, and social interaction	15 people with early stage of Alzheimer's disease living at home, >65 years	The ethnographic approach, interviews, observations, and field notes	Holding onto personal faith; seeking reassurance and hope; staying connected; effects of Alzheimer's disease on spirituality
Dalby et al. [11], UK	To understand the experience of spirituality in the context of living with dementia	6 people > 60 years, aware of the diagnosis of dementia	An exploratory study, semi-structured interview, IPA	Experience of faith; searching for meaning in dementia; changes and losses in the experience of the self; current pathways to spiritual connection and expression
Gardiner [24], USA	To describe the meaning of spirituality and religion, as experienced by older with Alzheimer's dementia	8 older adults with dementia	A Heideggerian interpretative method; interview each participant three times	Meaning from occupations; meaning from interactions with other people; meaning that organized religious and spiritual activities
MacKinlay [25], Australia	Examines spirituality and meaning in the experience of dementia of older Latvian residents	3 people with dementia living in a nursing home, MMSE scores between 18 and 20, 87–94 years	Grounded theory, in-depth interviews, small group work	Meaning in life; the need for relationship and connectedness, the participants' relationship with God and the ways participants responded to meaning through spiritual and religious practices

McGee and Myers [26], USA	To understand the impact and the spiritual dimensions of living with dementia	28 people with moderate Alzheimer's disease	Semi-structured interviews, constant comparative method	The Sacred Remains Important (the transcendent, the spiritual community, significant others); strengthening sacred relationships (identify roles, cultivate walk-alongside relationships, know the life story, create flexible and interactive spiritual experiences, normalize caring)
Phinney [27], USA	To uncover meaning in dementia	9 people with Alzheimer's disease	Interpretive phenomenological study; interview, field notes, observation	The meaning was unchanged; finding meaning in new ways of being
Snyder [28], USA	Researching the role of religion and spirituality	28 people with dementia	Interviews, documented verbatim quotes from clinicians, writings from persons with a disease	The role of religion or spirituality in finding meaning in dementia; the role of religion or spirituality in coping with the disease; the influence of dementia on religious or spiritual practices; the influence of dementia on faith
Sullivan and Beard [22], USA	The role of religion/spirituality in seniors dealing with Alzheimer's dementia	31 seniors diagnosed with early Alzheimer's disease	Individual and group interviews	Trust in God offers strength and hope; Never feeling alone/God as a friend; God helps with memory; keeping a positive attitude; contentment; the role of churches: social and interpersonal benefits

(continued)

Tab. 11.3 (continued)

References, country	Objective	Sample	Methodology	Identified themes
Trevitt and MacKinlay [23], Australia	Exploring spiritual reminiscence	16 residents with a diagnosis of dementia	In-depth interviews, small group discussion	Relationship and meaning (loneliness, family); attendance at worship (how these combine to give a sense of purpose), humour; insight into their illness and living circumstances
Trevitt and MacKinlay [29], Australia	To explore the religious and spiritual dimension in the life of older people living with dementia	22 participants with a diagnosis of dementia	Semi-structured interviews, observations, and small group sessions	Earliest memories of religious activities; relationship with God; meaning in life

Tab. 11.4: Overview of themes and subthemes.

Themes	Secondary subthemes	Primary subthemes
Spirituality as an inner source of power	Facing dementia	Unanswered questions
		Insights into the situation
		Hope and compassion
	Facing oneself	Loneliness
		Loss of self and identity
		Keeping contact with oneself
Spirituality as connectedness	Connections with others	Friendships
		Community and family
		Social isolation
	Connection with God	Belonging
		Deepening the relationship with God
		Religion and religious rites

of spirituality that offers older people with dementia, security and a sense of safety that, despite their illness, the core of who they are, will remain intact [11, 28].

Our results show that thinking about death is not related to being depressed. Older people with dementia can speak about death, calmly and without being stressed. Older people with dementia can talk openly about death, as they accept it as a normal process [23]. In addition to open talks about death, results show that older people with dementia are convinced that there is something inconceivable great that is waiting for them at the end of life [11, 23].

Facing oneself: Memories of personal loss from their early childhood, such as the loss of one's parents or siblings, are often accompanied by feelings of grief that surface daily. Therefore, older people with dementia feel lonely, despite being surrounded by people [23]. Older people with dementia are often willing to share their feelings of solitude, grief, and loneliness with other people with dementia; however, they usually have no one to turn to, which deepens their sadness [24, 25].

With their changed experience, there is a sense of loss in older people with dementia that affects their perception and experience, finding expression in spirituality [11]. People with dementia become frustrated due to their persistent memory problems since they can no longer depend on themselves, making them frustrated and they feel that they have lost their identity [24]. The results show that dementia takes away people's dignity and degrades them, which leads to despair [11]. We also find that their interaction with the environment changes due to the changed perceptions, which also causes various emotional responses, ranging from mild shocks and frustrations to deep feelings of sadness and anger [11].

Older people with dementia still feel much the same as before the onset of the illness, despite all the losses, not remembering everything and losing some of their knowledge and, consequently, having problems with everyday activities [27]. Therefore, it is also a reason why engaging with one's spirituality is essential [28]. Looking at oneself to connect with one's thoughts, one has to take time, all of which significantly impact their life [24]. Spiritual values are maintained despite their disease; however, the modes of expression change. Spiritual values preserve identity throughout the disease progression [11, 24, 25, 27].

Spirituality as connectedness

The second main theme, *Spirituality as connectedness,* was developed from two secondary subthemes: (1) connections with others; and (2) connection with God.

Connections with others: The data analysis shows that joint activities, conversations, relationships with friends, and socializing are critical elements of older people's spirituality with dementia [24, 26, 29]. Meeting friends, for instance, at religious rituals is, for some older people with dementia, the only way to maintain social contact [29].

In addition to friends, an essential reflection of spiritual life is the relationship and connection with family members and the community in which older people with dementia live [11, 22, 26]. Relationships and fostering connections with influential individuals, families, and the community represent a source of incentive and joy for older people with dementia, which is why they are an essential reflection of spirituality [26]. Interpersonal relations within the family are necessary because of the sense of connection and belonging they evoke [22]. They serve as support for older people dealing with dementia – an essential spiritual expression [11].

Often, older people who experience dementia avoid social contact because of the awareness of their cognitive decline, which can cause frustration and agitation [11, 26]. Sometimes, a complete break in social connections can happen [11]. We also find a decrease in their social contacts, mainly due to their limited ability to maintain interpersonal relationships and establish new relationships [28].

Connection with God: The importance of a sense of belonging to God and the church is emphasized by numerous studies [11, 15, 26, 29]. When going through difficult times, the connection to God is crucial as it helps overcome the fear of the future and offers a sense of security [26]. Participation in religious rites, such as singing at Mass, gives older people with dementia, a feeling that, despite their illness, they are worthy and still belong [15].

Their relationship with God is more than something ethereal and abstract. God is their friend who is intimately involved in their daily lives and is someone they can always connect with and turn to for support, advice, or a conversation. Some studies report that the disease intensified and deepened their connection with God [11, 22]. Their bond with God deepens because they seek and find solace in it, as they are sure that it is always there somewhere, can be counted on, and turned to when facing challenges with their memory. They often turn to God for help when searching for things or when they cannot remember something [22].

Some rites, such as prayer, church visits, or meditations, can deepen the contact with God [11, 15, 23], making it possible for older people with dementia to function normally [11, 23]. Faith is a constant that remains and deepens even in the face of the disease or appears because of it [11].

11.4 Discussion

In older people with dementia, spirituality plays a unique role. It is vital in their everyday lives since it enables them to develop the mechanisms they need to deal with and tackle dementia, and provides them the ability to find a new meaning, which affects the quality of their lives.

Therefore, spirituality permeates older people's lives, shaping their life paths and seems crucial in discovering inner strength in dealing with dementia and seeking new meaning in life . Our findings show that older people with dementia retain insights into their experience with spirituality. Deep inside, they are still the same people but are unable to and are incapable of expressing themselves in the same way as they could, before the disease. Spirituality is a way of manifesting the wholeness of that person living with dementia, helping them express themselves. Thus, this is an opportunity for their spiritual development and enrichment [11].

We found that spirituality enables older people with dementia to access their resources deep within their most profound, hidden powers [11, 27, 28]. Faith, hope, love, and compassion are essential factors that give a sense of security, power, and gratitude. In this search for their internal powers, they do not avoid talking about death and about end of life [23], which they perceive as something unimaginably grand, but at the same time, they see it as something that inspires hope and inner peace [11].

Hope is incredibly essential. It can make it easier for older people to cope with their loss of identity and deal with solitude, loneliness, and sadness, which they overcome by maintaining contact with their essence, their spirit. Hope is an essential inner factor of spirituality that is highlighted by many authors [15, 22, 27]. It refers to experiencing dementia, to the hope relating to the progression of the disease, the hope that they will be able to cope with the consequences of cognitive decline, and finally, the hope that death brings inner peace. Hope supports the course of the disease. It is reflected in a new attitude towards oneself, and the confirmation of one's values and the meaning of life. Older people with dementia understand spirituality by finding meaning in their disease and going through illness to life fulfilment.

It is also confirmed that older people with dementia often ask themselves questions such as: "Why I got dementia? Why right me? Will I manage? Why is this happening to me? What am I learning from this experience?" [11, 27, 28]. Such questions are frustrating [11], as they often remain unanswered or they raise a series of new issues that cannot be resolved [23, 27]. Such questions without the right answers make them vulnerable as they are aware that their lives are transient, and without spiritual care, they do not get the support they need and deserve. The spiritual needs of people with dementia must be understood. Indeed, the assessment of spiritual needs is crucial [30]. The researcher recommends a simple two-step approach by asking: "What is important to you right now?" and "How can we help?" [31].

This review's main finding is that relationships are critical in spirituality's role and meaning in people living with dementia. Relationships are a common denominator in many concepts of spirituality. These primarily relate to relationships with oneself, others, God, and nature. Relationships relate to hope and the meaning of life, and are shaped based on an individual's personal experience. Friends and family are crucial in maintaining interpersonal relationships [22, 24, 26]. People with dementia describe relationship with friends and family as a powerful reflection of spirituality. Maintaining relationships with friends and family is essential, mainly because of their fight with the frustration caused by the decline in cognitive functions. Maintaining contact, interpersonal relationships, and relationships with their partners imbue them with a sense of security and, at the same time, strengthens the family's connection, despite dementia. Therefore, nursing care should provide a safe environment where the older person with dementia feels safe and accepted despite his/her condition. In this respect, we agree with the other studies [23, 27] that relationships are essential elements of spirituality.

The connection with family and the relationship with God [32] are stressed as essential elements of spirituality in older people living with dementia. For some people with dementia, such a connection may be provided by the feeling of a link to the metaphysical [32]. Religious rituals, prayers, and meditations represent spiritual expression [15, 23]. Deepening relationships and faith in people with dementia can be understood as spirituality that remains intact despite the illness, which causes cognitive decline and loss. In this way, deepening and strengthening spirituality presents an inner force that gives older people with dementia the power to accept the disease and face the daily challenges.

This systematic review has some limitations. Some relevant literature may have been omitted, as we accessed only the English language selection. The fact that only studies with a qualitative research design were included is another limitation. Furthermore, the methodological quality of studies varied. The included studies were carried out in very different religious, cultural, and social environments, and all studies, except one, were conducted outside Europe.

11.5 Conclusion

This systematic review draws attention to the role and meaning of spirituality from the perspective of older people with dementia. The findings show the importance of spirituality as an inner source of power that gives people with dementia, the strength to face it, and highlights the role and meaning of connectedness with the self, others, and God. Friendships and relationships with family and the community are essential elements of spiritual life, and represent a source of incentive and joy for older people with dementia. The benefits of this review are, providing new insight into the role and meaning of spirituality as experienced by older people with dementia, and implementing spiritual care as an integral part of providing holistic person-centred care.

References

[1]   Blaser R, Berset J. Setting matters: Associations of nurses' attitudes towards people with dementia. Nurs Open, 2019, 6(1), 155–161.
[2]   Rognstad MK, Nåden D, Ulstein I, Kvaal K, Langhammer B, Sagbakken M. Behavioural disturbances in patients with frontotemporal lobe degeneration focusing on caregiver burden at home and in nursing homes. J Clin Nurs, 2020, 29(9–10), 1733–1743.
[3]   Aiken LH, Sermeus W, Van Den Heede K, Sloane DM, Busse R, McKee M, et al. Patient safety, satisfaction, and quality of hospital care: Cross sectional surveys of nurses and patients in 12 countries in Europe and the United States. BMJ, 2012, 344(2), e1717–e.
[4]   Scerri A, Innes A, Scerri C. Discovering what works well: Exploring quality dementia care in hospital wards using an appreciative inquiry approach. J Clin Nurs, 2015, 24(13–14), 1916–1925.
[5]   Toivonen K, Charalambous A, Suhonen R. Supporting spirituality in the care of older people living with dementia: A hermeneutic phenomenological inquiry into nurses' experiences. Scand J Caring Sci, 2018, 32(2), 880–888.
[6]   Suwa S, Yumoto A, Ueno M, Yamabe T, Hoshishiba Y, Sato M. Characteristics of care methods for daily life disabilities in Alzheimer's type dementia that respect autonomy and independence. Nurs Open, 2019, 6(3), 930–941.
[7]   Weathers E. What is spirituality? In: Timmins F, Caldeira S, eds. Spirituality in healthcare: Perspectives for innovative practice. Cham, Springer International Publishing, 2019, 1–22.
[8]   McSherry W, Jamieson S. An online survey of nurses' perceptions of spirituality and spiritual care. J Clin Nurs, 2011, 20(11–12), 1757–1767.
[9]   Veloza-Gómez M, Muñoz de Rodríguez L, Guevara-Armenta C, Mesa-Rodríguez S. The importance of spiritual care in nursing practice. J Holist Nurs, 2017, 35(2), 118–131.
[10] Powers BA, Watson NM. Spiritual nurturance and support for nursing home residents with dementia. Dementia, 2011, 10(1), 59–80.
[11] Dalby P, Sperlinger DJ, Boddington S. The lived experience of spirituality and dementia in older people living with mild to moderate dementia. Dementia, 2011, 11(1), 75–94.
[12] Cockell N, McSherry W. Spiritual care in nursing: An overview of published international research. J Nurs Manag, 2012, 20(8), 958–969.
[13] Daly L, Fahey-McCarthy E, Timmins F. The experience of spirituality from the perspective of people living with dementia: A systematic review and meta-synthesis. Dementia, 2019, 18(2), 448–470.

[14]   Agli O, Bailly N, Ferrand C. Spirituality and religion in older adults with dementia: A
        systematic review. Int Psychogeriatr, 2015, 27(5), 715–725.
[15]   Beuscher L, Grando VT. Using spirituality to cope with early-stage Alzheimer's disease. West J
        Nurs Res, 2009, 31(5), 583–598.
[16]   Kevern P. The spirituality of people with late-stage dementia: A review of the research
        literature, a critical analysis and some implications for person-centred spirituality and
        dementia care. Ment Health Relig Cult, 2015, 18(9), 765–776.
[17]   Thomas J, Harden A. Methods for the thematic synthesis of qualitative research in systematic
        reviews. BMC Med Res Methodol, 2008, 8(1), 45.
[18]   Sandelowski M, Barroso J, Voils CI. Using qualitative metasummary to synthesize qualitative
        and quantitative descriptive findings. Res Nurs Health, 2007, 30(1), 99–111.
[19]   Moher D, Shamseer L, Clarke M, Ghersi D, Liberati A, Petticrew M, et al. Preferred reporting
        items for systematic review and meta-analysis protocols (PRISMA-P) 2015 statement. Syst
        Rev, 2015, 4(1), 1.
[20]   Bettany-Saltikov J. How to do a systematic literature review in nursing: A step-by-step guide.
        Maidenhead. Open University Press, 2012.
[21]   Lockwood C, Munn Z, Porritt K. Qualitative research synthesis: Methodological guidance for
        systematic reviewers utilizing meta-aggregation. Int J Evid Based Healthc, 2015, 13(3), 179–187.
[22]   Sullivan SC, Beard RL. Faith and forgetfulness: The role of spiritual identity in preservation of
        self with Alzheimer's. J Relig Spiritual Aging, 2014, 26(1), 65–91.
[23]   Trevitt C, MacKinlay E. "I am just an ordinary person . . .": Spiritual reminiscence in older
        people with memory loss. J Relig Spiritual Aging, 2006, 18(2–3), 79–91.
[24]   Gardiner LB. The meaning of spirituality in elders with dementia. Marquette University, 2009.
[25]   MacKinlay E. Using spiritual reminiscence with a small group of Latvian residents with
        dementia in a nursing home: A multifaith and multicultural perspective. J Relig Spiritual
        Aging, 2009, 21(4), 318–329.
[26]   McGee JS, Myers D. Sacred relationships, strengthened by community, can help people with
        mild or early-stage Alzheimer's. Generations, 2014, 38(1), 61–67.
[27]   Phinney A. Horizons of meaning in dementia: Retained and shifting narratives. J Relig
        Spiritual Aging, 2011, 23(3), 254–268.
[28]   Snyder L. Satisfactions and challenges in spiritual faith and practice for persons with
        dementia. Dementia, 2003, 2(3), 299–313.
[29]   Trevitt C, MacKinlay E. 'Just because I can't remember . . .' religiousness in older people with
        dementia. J Relig Gerontol, 2004, 16(3–4), 109–121.
[30]   McSherry W, Boughey A, Attard J, eds. Enhancing nurses' and midwives' competence in
        providing spiritual care: through innovative education and compassionate care. Berlin/
        Heidelberg, Springer, 2021.
[31]   McSherry W, Ross L, Balthip K, Ross N, Young S. Spiritual assessment in healthcare: An
        overview of comprehensive, sensitive approaches to spiritual assessment for use within the
        interdisciplinary healthcare team. In: Timmins F, Caldeira S, eds. Spirituality in healthcare:
        Perspectives for innovative practice. Cham, Springer International Publishing, 2019, 39–54.
[32]   Rykkje LL, Eriksson K, Raholm MB. Spirituality and caring in old age and the significance of
        religion – a hermeneutical study from Norway. Scand J Caring Sci, 2013, 27(2), 275–284.

Dominika Vrbnjak, Majda Pajnkihar, John Nelson

12 Measuring the Caritas processes: Slovenian versions of the caring factor survey

Abstract: In Watson's Theory of Transpersonal Caring, it is mentioned that the concept of caring can be assessed by ten Caritas processes®. Initial psychometric evaluation of Slovenian instruments for measuring the Caritas process showed adequate psychometric properties. However, a further validation and testing the construct validity in a larger sample was suggested. Therefore, the study aimed to further evaluate the psychometrics of three Slovene versions of the Caring Factor Survey (CFS) among nursing staff. A cross-sectional study was carried out. A total of 1,295 nursing staff in 11 Slovenian hospitals were requested to take part in the study. Slovene version of the 20-item CFS-Care Provider Version, 10-item CFS-Caring of Manager, and 10-item CFS-Caring of Co-workers were used to collect data. Descriptive and inferential statistics were used. The study provided a shorter, valid, and reliable version of the CFS-Care Provider Version for Slovene hospital environments. The study also confirmed that the Slovene CFS for assessing the caring of managers and co-workers, as asserted in Watson's theory, are valid and reliable instruments. These instruments can be used for the evaluation of measuring caring in hospital settings.

Keywords: Psychometric evaluation, Item-reduction, Caring, Caritas processes

12.1 Introduction

Caring is an essential concept in nursing [1], with no simple definition [2]. It includes caring for self and for others [3], humanity, compassion, authenticity, promotion of well-being [2], and intimate interpersonal relationships [4]. There are several caring theories, including Jean Watson's Theory of Transpersonal Caring, which is most known and used worldwide in nursing practice, education, and research. The theory combines the "essence of contemporary nursing and wholeness of mind, body, and soul as person-centred transpersonal caring" [1].

Caring, as a latent construct, can be measured using formal measurement tools. Several instruments have been created to measure complex phenomena like caring [5–7]. Tools provide objective indicators to generate data on patients' and care providers' experience of caring [5]. Measuring caring can also contribute to empirical validation and refinement of theory, as understanding is sought of relationships between caring and healing outcomes [5]. Researchers developed more than 20 tools to assess caring and more than six tools to measure caring, from the original Watson's

Theory of Transpersonal Caring and her ten caring factors [8]. Watson refined her theory, and Caritas processes have been proposed [9, 10]. However, none of the developed instruments had incorporated the contemporary concept of the Ten Caritas processes, which combines caring, love, and self-caring practices [11] and include embracing loving-kindness, inspiring faith-hope, trusting transpersonal, nurturing relationships, forgiving all, deepening creative self, balancing learning, co-creating Caritas field, ministering humanity, and open infinity [9].

Therefore, the Caring Factor Survey – CFS, an instrument that measures Ten Caritas processes, has been developed [12]. Derivation tools within this study aimed to measure the experience of Caritas processes provided by care providers (CFS-CP) [13], care managers (CFS-CM) [14], and co-workers (CFS-CC) [15].

The original CFS CP was developed and tested as a 20-item scale, with two items for each Caritas process [13]. Further psychometric evaluation resulted in a reduced 10-item questionnaire [16]. Other versions, CFS–CM and CFS–CC were developed as 10-item scales. All three versions implement a 7-item Likert scale (1 – strongly disagree, 7 – strongly agree).

Initial psychometric evaluation of Slovenian tools for measuring the Caritas processes showed acceptable psychometrical properties [4, 17]. Nonetheless, further validation and testing of construct validity in a larger sample size were suggested.

12.2 Aim

To evaluate the construct validity and internal consistency of the CFS for care providers, managers, and co-workers among Slovene nursing staff. The authors of this study also sought to evaluate the item reduction from 20 to 10 items for CFS-CP and the discriminant validity to measure the Watson's Caritas processes.

12.3 Methods

The study's results were based on secondary data analysis from a cross-sectional study [4].

12.3.1 Setting and sample

A convenience sample of nursing staff working on surgical and internal medicine wards in eleven healthcare institutions in Slovenia was included. Inclusion criteria were nurses and nursing assistants employed by the hospitals. The exclusion criteria were nursing staff like nurse managers, who were not involved in patient care. Of

1,295 administered surveys, 790 were returned (61% response rate) [4]. The sample size exceeded the recommendation of 10 participants per scale item [18], and the recommendation by Tabachnik and Fidel, who suggest that a sample of 400 is adequate for factor analysis [19].

12.3.2 Data collection and ethics

Three different versions of the CFS, CFS-CP [16], CFS-CM [14], and CFS-CC [15] were used to measure the Caritas processes. The process of developing Slovenian versions of CFS can be found elsewhere [4, 17].

Data was gathered between October 2015 and March 2016. The researcher, nursing manager or study-designated coordinator distributed surveys at the wards on day shifts. Respondents were provided two weeks to respond and submit their survey. The return of a completed survey was considered as willingness to take part in the research. Permissions from the included healthcare institutions and the National Medical Ethics Committee (No. 127/07/14) were sought. Participation in the survey was voluntary. Anonymity was assured as respondents returned the completed surveys in sealed envelopes or boxes, with no identifying information.

12.3.3 Data analysis

Descriptive statistics from each of the CFS tools are presented with mean values and standard deviations. Higher scores indicate perceptions of more caring [20]. Principal component analysis, oblique rotation, and Eigenvalues greater than 1.0 for factor loading with Keiser-Meyer-Olkin (KMO) for model fit, desiring at least 0.85 [19], were used to evaluate the construct validity of the selected instruments, and to reduce the 20–item CFS–CP to 10 items. Bartlett's test of sphericity was also used to determine the appropriateness of PCA [21]. Cronbach's alpha (acceptable above 0.7) and corrected item-total correlations (acceptable above 0.3) were utilized to evaluate internal consistency [22]. Discriminant validity of the CFS-CC and CFS-CM are presented elsewhere [4], while the discriminant validity of the CFS-CP tool was tested within this current study. The variations of mean scores were evaluated for all CFS-CP items to identify variations. CFS-CP differences between both wards were analysed with the Mann–Whitney U-test.

12.4 Results

Most respondents were female ($n = 684$, 87.50%) nursing assistants ($n = 378$, 51.10%) who worked in the surgical ($n = 507$, 64.20%) or internal medicine wards ($n = 278$, 35.40%), and reported working a mean of 16.19 years (SD = 11.06). The average age was 37.58 (SD = 10.02). The highest mean for all items was found for the Caritas process, Teaching and learning, while the lowest was for Miracles for CFS-CC and CFS-CM. Decision-making was found with the lowest mean score for CFS-CP. Descriptive statistics of the 20-item CFS-CP, 10-item CFS-CM, and the 10-item CFS-CC are shown in Tab. 12.1.

Tab. 12.1: Descriptive statistics of CFs tool.

Caritas process	20-item CFS-CP			10-item CFS-CM			10-item CFS-CC		
	n	M	SD	n	M	SD	n	M	SD
1 Practice loving-kindness	748	5.92	.30	744	5.34	1.50	748	4.93	1.45
2 Decision-making	745	5.39	.39	746	5.30	1.48	748	5.00	1.42
3 Instil faith and hope	746	6.00	.27	747	5.31	1.45	748	5.08	1.34
4 Teaching and learning	745	**6.05**	.21	747	**5.44**	1.46	752	**5.34**	1.23
5 Spiritual beliefs and practices	746	5.96	.23	746	4.97	1.69	743	4.99	1.42
6 Holistic care	742	5.95	.26	746	5.17	1.59	746	5.05	1.38
7 Helping and trusting relationship	747	5.84	.39	746	5.27	1.56	747	5.25	1.30
8 Healing environment	744	5.72	.38	745	4.97	1.64	743	5.03	1.41
9 Promote expression of feelings	742	6.00	.27	747	5.17	1.65	748	4.98	1.45
10 Miracles	739	5.56	.37	738	4.88	1.67	739	4.77	1.53
Total	750	5.84	.78	755	5.18	1.40	752	5.04	1.24

CFS-CC, Caring Factor Survey-Caring for Co-workers; CFS-CM, Caring Factor Survey-Caring of Manager; CFS-CP, Caring Factor Survey-Care Provider version; *M*, *mean*; *n*, number; SD, standard deviation

To evaluate construct validity, we tested two models of CFS–CC. Model 1 included 10–items from the original short version in English: items 1, 4, 7, 8, 9, 10, 13, 16, 17, 20 [11]. Model 2 included 10 items (items 2, 3, 5, 6, 11, 12, 14, 15, 18, 19), not in the original English short version. For Model 1, items loaded into one component, with factor loadings between 0.54 and 0.83, and explained 58% of the data variance. The KMO for Model 1 was .92 with the Bartlett's test of sphericity, $\chi^2 = 4078.78$, df = 45, $p \leq 0.001$. Model 2 items were loaded into two separate components, with factor loadings between 0.48 and 0.75, and explained 53% data variance. KMO for Model 2 was 0.88 with the Bartlett's test of sphericity being $\chi^2 = 4,512.57$, df = 45, $p \leq 0.001$. Cronbach's alpha was 0.90 for Model 1 and 0.89 for Model 2. The corrected item-total correlations ranged from 0.46 to 0.78.

For CFS-CM, all 10 items loaded as a single factor. Factor loadings ranged from 0.76 to 0.85 and explained 78% of the data variance. KMO was 0.91. Bartlett's test of sphericity showed acceptable values ($\chi^2 = 9,717.70$, df = 45, $p \leq 0.001$). Cronbach's alpha was 0.96. The corrected item-total correlations ranged from 0.76 to 0.9.

For CFS-CC, all 10 items loaded as a single factor, with factor loadings from 0.72 to 0.86, and explained 80% of variance in the data. The KMO was 0.92 and the Bartlett's test of sphericity also showed acceptable values ($\chi^2 = 9{,}209.15$, df = 45, $p \leq 0.001$). Cronbach's alpha was 0.97. The corrected item-total correlations ranged from 0.81 to 0.91.

Table 12.2 shows descriptive statistics and discriminant validity analysis for the reduced 10-item CFS-CP. Statistically significant differences between both wards were detected for four items (items 8, 10, 13, 17).

Tab. 12.2: Descriptive statistics and discriminant validity for the reduced 10-item CFS-CP.

Caritas process	Reduced 10-item CFS-CP	All	Surgical wards	Internal medicine wards	
		M (SD)	M (SD)	M (SD)	p-Value
1 Practice loving-kindness	Item 1	5.85 (0.75)	5.84 (1.13)	5.86 (1.08)	0.99
2 Decision-making	Item 4	5.51 (1.12)	5.48 (1.20)	5.57 (1.23)	0.159
3 Instil faith and hope	Item 7	6.04 (1.22)	6.09 (0.84)	5.95 (1.03)	0.162
4 Teaching and learning	Item 8	6.01 (0.92)	6.09 (0.80)	5.86 (1.03)	0.008*
5 Spiritual beliefs and practices	Item 9	6.10 (0.95)	6.17 (0.80)	5.99 (1.05)	0.109
6 Holistic care	Item 16	6.04 (0.95)	6.08 (0.92)	5.96 (0.99)	0.118
7 Helping and trusting relationship	Item 13	5.95 (0.96)	6.03 (0.89)	5.80 (1.04)	0.005*
8 Healing environment	Item 10	5.91 (0.98)	5.99 (0.87)	5.77 (1.14)	0.039*
9 Promote expression of feelings	Item 17	6.00 (0.95)	6.07 (0.89)	5.89 (0.99)	0.019*
10 Miracles	Item 20	5.71 (0.93)	6.08 (1.20)	5.67 (1.3)	0.607

CFS-CP, Caring Factor Survey-Care Provider Version; M, mean; SD, standard deviation; p, statistical significance; *, statistical significance at ≤0.05.

12.5 Discussion

Our study aimed to evaluate the psychometric properties of the CFS for care providers, managers, and co-workers, as perceived by the nursing staff.

The mean values for CFS-CP, CFS-CM, and CFS-CC were all above 4.0, meaning that caring was perceived, overall as average [7]. Nursing staff evaluated themselves as the most caring, while the caring of their manager and colleagues were evaluated with slightly lower scores. Results were consistent with what is found in literature, as nurses tend to describe themselves as caring [23]. The results of this study's when compared with the American CFS-CP results reveal these scores to be equal or slightly lower. Mean values in similar studies were found to be 5.0 [24] or above 6.0 [25]. We found the highest mean for the Caritas process, Teaching and learning. The lowest score was found for Miracles for CFS-CM and CFS-CC. Allowing miracles and mysteries in nursing is not typical of the Slovenian environment, where the biomedical model still dominates [26]. Interestingly, decision-making was found to be perceived as the worst for CFS-CP. Results suggest that improvements are needed in nursing and in healthcare teams with respect to problem solving and decision-making. In a similar American research, teaching and learning [24], practising loving-kindness [25], and miracles [13] were rated with the highest mean scores, while creating a healing environment [13, 24] and decision-making [25] were rated with the lowest mean values [25].

We have validated the construct of Caritas processes for the reduced 10-item CFS-CP, CFS-CM, and CFS-CC. Results of the Bartlett's test of sphericity and the KMO confirmed the appropriateness of PCA. All items in the CFS-CP Model 1 for CFS-CM and CFS-CC were loaded as a single factor, suggesting that items belong to the same construct. A shorter instrument is less time-consuming to complete, which could reduce the reluctance to participate in research and increase the response rate. Instruments were found to be reliable, as Cronbach's values were greater than 0.70. Considering the satisfactory discriminant validity, CFS-CP can be helpful for assessing differences in caring perceptions among different groups.

Limitations of our study include convenience sampling and inclusion of only two wards in hospital settings. Criterion validity and retest reliability should be evaluated in further research, which should also include other settings.

12.6 Conclusion

The study found that the Slovene version of the reduced construct to measure the Caritas processes from the care providers' perspective, CFS-CP, CFS-CM, and CFS-CC are valid and reliable tools that can be further used in hospitals. These tools enable further research of the links between caring perceptions, and patient and organizational outcomes.

References

[1] Pajnkihar M, McKenna HP, Stiglic G, Vrbnjak D. Fit for practice: Analysis and evaluation of Watson's theory of human caring. Nurs Sci Q, 2017, 30(3), 243–252.
[2] Cook LB, Peden A. Finding a focus for nursing: The caring concept. ANS Adv Nurs Sci, 2017, 40(1), 12–23.
[3] Pajnkihar M. Theory development for nursing in Slovenia [PhD thesis]. Manchester: University of Manchester, Faculty of Medicine, Dentistry, Nursing and Pharmacy, 2003.

[4]   Vrbnjak D. Caring for patient and safety in medication administration in nursing. Maribor, University of Maribor, 2017.

[5]   Watson J. Assessing and measuring caring in nursing and health sciences. Watson's caring science guide. 3rd ed. New York, Springer Publishing Company, LLC, 2019.

[6]   Watson J. Assessing and measuring caring in nursing and health science. 2nd ed. New York, Springer Publishing Company, 2009.

[7]   Nelson J, Watson J. Measuring caring: International research on Caritas as healing. New York, Springer Publishing Company, 2012.

[8]   Sitzman K, Watson J. Assessing and measuring caring in nursing and health sciences. 3rd ed. New York, Springer Publishing Company, 2019.

[9]   Watson J. Unitary caring science: The philosophy and praxis of nursing. Louisville, University Press of Colorado, 2018.

[10]   Watson J. Nursing: The philosophy and science of caring (revised edition). Boulder, CO, University Press of Colorado, 2008.

[11]   Nelson J, Watson J, Health I. Development of the Caring Factor Survey (CFS)m an instrument to measure patient's perception of caring. In: Sitzman K, Watson J, Eds. Assessing and measuring caring in nursing and health sciences Watson's caring science guide. New York, Springer Publishing Company, LLC, 2019, 271–279.

[12]   Persky GJ, Nelson J, Watson J, Bent K. Creating a profile of a nurse effective in caring. Nurs Adm Q, 2008, 32(1), 15–20.

[13]   Johnson J. Creation of the Caring Factor Survey-Care Provider Version (CFS-CPV). In: Nelson J, Watson J, Eds. Measuring caring, International research on caritas as healing. New York, Springer Publishing Company, LLC, 2012, 40–46.

[14]   Olender L, Phifer S. Development of the Caring Factor Survey-Caring of Manager (CFS-CM). In: Nelson J, Watson J, Eds. Measuring caring, International research on caritas as healing. New York, Springer Publishing Company, 2012, 57–63.

[15]   Lawerence I, Kear M. The practice of loving kindness to self and others as perceived by nurses and patients in the cardiac interventional unit (CIU). In: Nelson J, Watson J, Eds. Measuring caring, International research on caritas as healing. New York, Springer Publishing Company, LLC, 2012.

[16]   DiNapoli PP, Nelson J, Turkel M, Watson J. Measuring the Caritas processes: Caring factor survey. Ijhc, 2010, 14(3), 15–20.

[17]   Vrbnjak D, Pahor D, Štiglic G, Pajnkihar M. Content validity and internal reliability of Slovene version of medication administration error survey. Obzornik Zdravstvene Nege, 2016, 50(1), 20–40.

[18]   Polit D, Beck C. Nursing research: Generating and assessing evidence for nursing practice. 9th ed. Philadelphia, Wolters Kluwer, Lippincott Williams & Wilkins, 2012.

[19]   Tabachnick B, Fidell L. Using multivariate statistics. 7th ed. Pearson, 2018.

[20]   Nelson J, Thiel L, Hozak MA, Thomas ST. Item reduction of the caring factor survey–care provider version, an instrument specified to measure Watson's 10 processes of caring. Int J Hum Caring, 2016, 3, 123–128.

[21]   Nunnaly J, Bernstein IH. Psychometric theory. 3rd ed. New Yirj, McGraw-Hill, 1994.

[22]   Polit DF, Beck CT. Nursing research: Generating and assessing evidence for nursing practice. 10th ed. Philadelphia, PA, Lippincott Williams & Wilkins, 2017.

[23]   Ousey K, Johnson M. Being a real nurse – concepts of caring and culture in the clinical areas. Nurse Educ Pract, 2007, 7(3), 150–155.

[24] Testerman RL. Preceptor caring attributes as perceived by graduate nurses. In: Nelson J, Watson J, Eds. Measuring caring, International research on Caritas as healing. New York, Springer Publishing Company, 2012.

[25] Hozak MA, Brennan M. Caring at the core: Maximizing the likelihood that a caring moment will occur. In: Nelson J, Watson J, Eds. Measuring caring international research on caritas as healing. New York, Springer Publishing Company, 2012.

[26] Pajnkihar M, Stiglic G, Vrbnjak D. The concept of Watson's carative factors in nursing and their (dis)harmony with patient satisfaction. PeerJ, 2017, 5, e2940.

Majda Pajnkihar, Dominika Vrbnjak, Gregor Štiglic,
Primož Kocbek, Marlaine Smith, Kasandra Musović

13 Fit for practice: assessing faculty nurse caring behaviours

Abstract: A theory, knowledge, and evidence-based curriculum where caring is the central focus of the discipline of nursing provides a foundation to guide the nursing profession. Positive faculty caring, role modelling, and creating caring environments enhance students' caring behaviours and values about caring. Caring outcomes in practice depend on learning and teaching processes; therefore, nurses' caring views mainly originate from nursing education. What is taught is as important as how it is taught. Nurse educators have a crucial role in creating a caring environment, modelling caring, and including caring in a nursing curriculum. Even so, there are restricted studies investigating faculty caring behaviours. Therefore, this study explored student nurses' perceptions of faculty caring behaviours. A cross-sectional study including 192 nursing students from Slovenia was conducted in April 2019. Data were collected using Caring Assessment Tool – Educational Version (CAT-edu), a 5-level Likert scale with a score ranging from 94 to 740 (least to most caring). The CAT-edu instrument was developed initially by Duffy and is based on Watson's Theory of Human Caring. Each item or several items together correspond to and reflect concepts of Watson's theory. Data were analysed using descriptive statistics and one-way ANOVA with the Tukey honest significant difference post-hoc test. The highest mean CAT-edu score was measured in the third-year students ($M = 324.6$, $SD = 46.5$), followed by first-year students ($M = 301.8$, $SD = 38.3$) and second-year students ($M = 285.3$, $SD = 43.8$). One-way ANOVA results show the statistically significant difference among students from different years of study ($F(2,188) = 14.06$, $p < 0.001$). Post-hoc testing confirms the difference between first- and third-year students ($p = 0.020$), second- and third-year students ($p < 0.001$), but not between first- and second-year students ($p = 0.084$). Caring is a foundation for implementing systematic, holistic, and individual patient care and developing human, professional, and equal interpersonal relationships. Assessing students' perceptions of faculty caring can provide important information about the educational program's structure and processes and help understand students' way of learning how to care for themselves and patients. Forming a positive, caring relationship between faculty and nursing students can create caring attributes in students. This study suggests some differences in incorporating caring into nursing curriculum and fostering caring and supporting caring behaviours by nurse educators. Despite limitations such as sample size, results can contribute to the body of caring knowledge. Results can be used in creating a caring environment, curriculum, and development of

Acknowledgment: The authors acknowledge student nurses who participated in this study.

effective strategies so that students will be fit to practice caring. Nurse educators can understand caring behaviours and form their role as caring nurse educators. Providing more efficient teaching/learning caring ensures safe, quality nursing care for the patients and nurses' work satisfaction.

Keywords: caring, faculty caring, student nurse

13.1 Introduction

Caring is a core value of nursing [1–10]. Caring has a positive effect on patients, nurses [11, 12], and organizations [13, 14] and has a significant influence on nursing care quality and safety of the patients [15–17]. Caring is an anticipated competency of nursing students [18–21]. There are inconsistencies and a lack of understanding of what caring means in nursing education. Different authors discuss caring and its importance to nursing education. However, all agree that their education affects nurses' perception of caring [22, 23].

Teaching caring behaviours should be taught through caring interactions with faculty [24]. The transition of caring into nursing practice is conditioned by its nurture in nursing education [25, 26]. The "what" that is taught is as important as "how" it is taught [27]. It is essential to create caring environments during the educational process and role model caring relationships [28]. Nursing curricula based on theory, knowledge, and evidence, where caring is the principal focus of the discipline, could provide a basis to direct the nursing profession [29]. Jean Watson's Theory of Human Caring supports and enhances nursing education [30], research, and practice [20, 31, 32] by highlighting and placing caring in the centre. Undergraduate and postgraduate nursing has been based on nursing theories; however, not well around caring theories. Consequently, this can have a toll on the nursing discipline [32].

Some nursing faculties pay more attention to caring in education than others [20, 32, 33]. Although nursing models are slowly being incorporated, the biomedical model in nursing can still be observed [32]. Several studies show that students do not quite understand what caring is and perceive caring in an instrumental manner [34–36]. An international cross-cultural study showed that students, who were taught caring theories, scored the highest on expressive dimensions of caring values compared to those whose faculties did not implement caring theories in their curriculum [35]. However, caring perceptions seem to vary according to the year of study [35, 37]. Nurse educators have an essential role in modelling caring in nursing education [38, 39]; thus, their caring behaviours positively influence students' caring behaviours [40]. There are several studies that focused on caring in nursing education. Nursing students feel that the faculty has role-modelled caring behaviours and have experienced and developed caring relationships during education. The findings also emphasize the necessity of developing the caring model in nursing education [41]. Another study demonstrated the importance of connecting caring theory to caring practice. Implementing caring in the nursing education curriculum facilitates the students' understanding of caring in clinical nursing situations and supports their growth in their understanding of caring through modelling [42].

Empirical evidence of the value of environments based on theory-based behaviours has never been more critically important [43]. Assessing students' perceptions of faculty caring can provide important information about the educational program's structure and processes [44] and can help understand student nurses' way of learning how to care [38, 45]. Therefore, this research explored nursing students' perceptions of faculty caring behaviours.

13.2 Methods

13.2.1 Study design

The study implemented a descriptive cross-sectional design.

13.2.2 Setting and participants

The study included 192 undergraduate nursing students in Slovenia from a faculty that implemented Watson's theory in the nursing study programs. In Slovenia, the nursing education program lasts 3 years (180 ECTS credits). The convenience sampling method was used to recruit participants. The required sample size was calculated for population data, 95% confidence level, and 5% margin of error [46]. The minimum sample size satisfying these criteria was calculated ($n = 186$). We have included both full- and part-time male or female nursing students attending first, second, or third year of studies. Before data collection, ethical approval was obtained from the institutional ethics committee.

13.2.3 Data collection and questionnaire

Data were collected in April 2019. The questionnaires were delivered to students while in the classrooms.

The first part of the questionnaire collected brief demographic data (sex, age, year of study, type of study). Next, the data was collected using the Caring Assessment Tool – Educational Version (CAT-edu) with permission from the author (License #001018). The tool has 94 items designed to capture students' perceptions of faculty nurse caring behaviours. The CAT-edu instrument was developed initially by Duffy in 1997 as an adaptation of the original Caring Assessment Tool (CAT) and is based on Jean Watson's theoretical framework. Each item or several items correspond to and reflect a "carative factor" and is assigned a Likert-type closed-response score measuring the frequency with which each behaviour occurs during a students' learning experience from 1 (never) to 5 (always); thus, the score has a possible range from 94 to 470. Several items (21) are worded negatively and/or overlap with other items; they were intentionally designed to minimize the chance of error or careless responding. Items numbered 4, 8, 13, 18, 27, 36, 38, 42, 44, 46, 51, 59, 62, 69, 74, 75, 80, 83, 85, 88, and 94 are such items. Those items were refactored inversely prior to the analysis. Individual item scores are summed up, giving us a total score that can be categorized from low to high caring. In the original version, Cronbach's coefficient alpha was 0.98 [47]. Alpha internal consistency reliability was measured at 0.97. The instrument was translated into Slovene language using back-translation as a gold standard for providing semantic equivalence [48]. Our Slovene version of the CAT-edu questionnaire in this study resulted in Cronbach's coefficient alpha of 0.75.

13.2.4 Statistical analysis

Data were analysed using descriptive statistics and one-way ANOVA with Tukey's honest significant difference (HSD) post-hoc test for pairwise comparisons. Furthermore, a one-way ANOVA test based on the year of study was performed with a corresponding post-hoc Tukey HSD test to evaluate the difference between the 2 years of study; in both cases, the average values of the instrument (CAT-edu) were compared. Additionally, mean values for each CAT-edu component by the year of study were compared with a one-factor ANOVA with a post-hoc Tukey HSD test to evaluate the difference between 2 years of study. A standard significance level of $\alpha = 0.05$ was used [49].

In 34 (17.7%) cases, at least one estimate was missing, and this would mean, for example, that even though the other 93 claims were evaluated, CAT-edu could not be calculated in this case. Therefore, we decided to impute the missing data using the method of K-nearest neighbour, where missing values are determined from the values of similar adjacent variables. Given that we impute data with the Likert scale, the recommendation [50] is to take the square root of the number of responses without missing values (158); in our case, that was 13. Data were analysed using R statistical software version 4.1.1 [51].

13.3 Results

A total of 192 undergraduate nursing students participated in the study, with at least 1 answer missing in 34 (17.7%) cases. Furthermore, in the assumptions for the one-way ANOVA, we observed that there was one solitary ("extremely" low-value "CAT-edu") that was removed from further analysis ($n = 191$), which is described in more detail further. The students were mostly female (85.9%, $n = 164$), enrolled full-time (96.3%, $n = 184$) in the study program and were on average 21.1 (SD = 2.9) years. Fifty (26.2%) first-year nursing students, 84 (44.0%) second-year nursing students, and 57 (29.8%) third-year nursing students were surveyed. A review of mean values by the year of study showed that the highest CAT-edu average was in third-year students with 326.7 (SD = 48.3), followed by first year with 302.8 (SD = 39.8) and second year with 285.9 (SD = 45.7) (Tab. 13.1 and Fig. 13.1).

Tab. 13.1: Average values and standard deviation of CAT-edu values according to the year of study.

Year of study	n	M	SD
First year	50	302.8	39.8
Second year	84	285.9	45.7
Third year	57	326.76	48.3

M, mean; n, number of participants; SD, standard deviation.

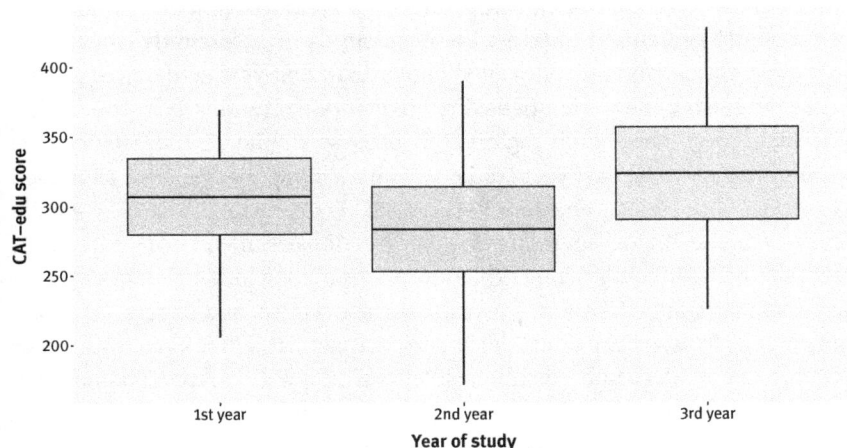

Fig. 13.1: CAT-edu quantile graphs according to the year of study.

The results of the one-way ANOVA show that there is a significant statistical difference between the years of study according to CAT-edu ($F(2,188) = 13.92$, $p < 0.001$). Tukey's post-hoc HSD shows that there is a statistical difference in the students' perception of faculty caring between first and third year (difference 23.9, $p = 0.0187$, higher in third year compared to first year) and between second and third year (difference 40.8, $p < 0.001$, higher in third year compared to second year), but not between first and second year (difference −16.9, $p = 0.092$). If, instead of the standard degree characteristic $\alpha = 0.05$, we take the degree characteristic 0.10, we notice that there is also a statistical difference between the first and second year of study.

Table 13.2 presents the results of individual items of the students' perceptions of faculty caring. The statement "answer my questions" ($M = 4.16$), "respect me" ($M = 4.09$), "look me in the eyes when they talk to me" ($M = 4.00$), and "don't want to talk to me" ($M = 3.96$) were rated the highest among all years. Because of the high number of items (94), we have decided to present only the most significant ones ($p < 0.001$).

13.4 Discussion

We have examined first-, second-, and third-year nursing students' perceptions of faculty caring. The study results showed that third-year students compared to first and second year have the highest CAT-edu score, meaning that the third-year students' perceptions of faculty nurse caring behaviours were the highest. The included Slovenian faculty has incorporated Watson's theory [17]. It is introduced to students in their first year of study and is nurtured during their clinical practice, which may influence students' perception of patient and faculty caring. Similarly, in a study done in Slovenia, third-year students scored higher than first-year students regarding caring behaviours using the Caring Behaviors Inventory instrument [52]. The similar results can be argued that similar regions can possess similar characteristics [53]. However, in a similar study, first-year students without clinical experience expressed higher agreement with caring behaviour items, which is interesting since they are the most vulnerable in the clinical environment [54]. Nevertheless, their strong agreement may reflect their beliefs about nursing [55]. Perceptions among nursing students probably differ, given different education, curricula, societal values, and culture [35, 56].

The statement "answer my questions", "respect me", and "look me in the eyes when they talk to me" were rated the highest among all 3 years. Caring communication skills and respect are essential characteristics of faculty caring behaviour that affect students' learning environment [57]. In another study, students ranked faculty characteristics in online caring rank providing timely communication the highest [58]. Jones et al. define caring as "intentional communication and actions designed to meet students' actual and potential needs for human connection, learning, support, and respect" [59, 60]. Our results also align with other studies that

Tab. 13.2: The results of individual items of students' perceptions of faculty caring according to the year of study (in descending order according to the average of all years).

No.	Statement	Average (all years)		First year	Second year	Third year	One-way ANOVA	Tukey's HSD
		M	SD	M(SD)	M(SD)	M(SD)		
48	Question me about my past experiences in nursing.	3.66	1.01	3.76 (1.0)	3.36 (1.01)	4.02 (0.9)	8.118 (p < 0.001)	Third > second
15	Support me with my beliefs.	3.39	0.86	3.52 (0.91)	3.11 (0.76)	3.68 (0.83)	9.263 (p < 0.001)	Second < first, third > second
11	Use my name when they talk to me.	3.37	1.23	3.76 (1.1)	2.9 (1.25)	3.7 (1.09)	11.85 (p < 0.001)	Second < first, third > second
65	Make me feel as comfortable as possible.	3.33	0.99	3.46 (1.01)	2.95 (0.88)	3.77 (0.93)	13.877 (p < 0.001)	Second < first, third > second
16	Help me to believe in myself.	3.29	0.98	3.42 (0.97)	3 (0.93)	3.6 (0.94)	7.425 (p < 0.001)	Second < first, third > second
84	Help me achieve my career goals.	3.20	0.96	3.1 (0.84)	2.98 (0.98)	3.61 (0.9)	8.508 (p < 0.001)	Third > first, third > second
14	Seem interested in me.	3.15	0.93	3.22 (0.93)	2.86 (0.87)	3.53 (0.87)	9.92 (p < 0.001)	Third > second
77	Keep me challenged.	3.06	0.91	2.88 (0.9)	2.9 (0.79)	3.44 (0.98)	7.682 (p < 0.001)	Third > first, third > second
43	Accept what I say, even when it is negative.	3.04	0.89	3.06 (0.79)	2.79 (0.89)	3.4 (0.86)	8.8 (p < 0.001)	Third > second
87	Understand my unique situation.	3.01	0.93	2.88 (0.75)	2.77 (0.96)	3.47 (0.87)	11.436 (p < 0.001)	Third > first, third > second

(continued)

Tab. 13.2 (continued)

No.	Statement	Average (all years)		First year	Second year	Third year	One-way ANOVA	Tukey's HSD
		M	SD	M(SD)	M(SD)	M(SD)		
73	Make me feel secure regarding my performance in school.	2.96	1.05	2.92 (0.94)	2.67 (0.99)	3.44 (1.07)	10.16 ($p < 0.001$)	Third > first, third > second
93	Show respect for those things that have meaning for me.	2.95	1.03	2.9 (1.04)	2.65 (0.91)	3.42 (1.03)	10.413 ($p < 0.001$)	Third > first, third > second
39	Encourage me to talk about whatever is on my mind.	2.79	1.02	2.52 (0.95)	2.63 (0.99)	3.25 (0.99)	9.16 ($p < 0.001$)	Third > first, third > second
81	Help me feel less worried.	2.75	1.08	2.7 (0.95)	2.39 (1.03)	3.33 (1.02)	14.863 ($p < 0.001$)	Third > first, third > second
54	Help me understand my feelings.	2.66	1.06	2.72 (0.99)	2.35 (1.04)	3.07 (1.02)	8.731 ($p < 0.001$)	Third > second
92	Helps me cope with the stress of my work.	2.62	1.03	2.58 (0.93)	2.33 (0.91)	3.09 (1.12)	10.079 ($p < 0.001$)	Third > first, third > second
76	Make sure I have time out for my own needs.	2.59	1.13	2.54 (1.01)	2.19 (1.02)	3.23 (1.12)	16.651 ($p < 0.001$)	Third > first, third > second
90	Knows what is important to me	2.56	1.09	2.54 (1.03)	2.27 (1.05)	3 (1.09)	8.062 ($p < 0.001$)	Third > second
72	Spend time with me.	2.31	1.11	2.46 (1.03)	1.98 (0.96)	2.68 (1.26)	8.01 ($p < 0.001$)	Second < first, third > second

M, mean; no., statement number; p, statistical significance at < 0.05; SD, standard deviation for mean.

one of desired faculty caring behaviours is "answering student questions patiently, directly, and respectfully" [60]. It appears that communication and respect are linked and desired faculty caring behaviour. Interestingly, "don't want to talk to me" is also highly rated. This item and its high rank do not match the previously mentioned items. We could assume that some students may be frustrated by the unavailability of the nurse educators. Communication and communication skills play an essential role in nursing education and practice [61]. Poor communication skills can lead to students lacking motivation, disliking faculty, and believing they cannot accomplish themselves [62]. The statement "spend time with me" was, intriguingly, rated the lowest, congruent with the highly rated item "don't want to talk to me". Students' perception on faculty caring impacts their academic performance. The faculty's positive outlook and compassion towards students are associated with nursing students' improved academic performance. Faculty–student interactions and student outcomes in nursing practice are shaped by the conditions in the learning environment [63].

13.4.1 Limitations

Several limitations should be considered when interpreting our results. Convenience sampling allows limited generalization of the results. The data were collected at one faculty in Slovenia; therefore, it cannot represent all the population of nursing students in Slovenia. It is impossible to establish casual relations with a cross-sectional design. Hence, longitudinal studies would be preferred.

13.5 Conclusion

Despite our study limitations, it provided an overview of students' perceptions of faculty caring behaviours. Third-year nursing students rated faculty caring behaviours as the highest compared to first- and second-year students. This could be due to their long relationship with the faculty, and they have already been exposed to clinical practice and caring theories. Some students rated items "answer my questions", "respect me", and "look me in the eyes when they talk to me" the highest, which stresses the importance of communication and respect between faculty and students. On the other hand, students feel that their teachers do not spend enough time or talk to them as they wish they would. Similarly, in nursing practice, the patients need to communicate with health professionals and want their real caring presence. The results show that nursing education should emphasize incorporating caring theories and facilitating the caring relationship between faculty and students. Creating a caring academic environment will allow the transition of caring behaviours into nursing practice, where the nurses and patients will be supported, as well as patients' families.

Funding: The authors received no financial support for this study's authorship and/or publication.

Conflict of interests: The authors declared no potential conflicts of interest with respect to the authorship and/or publication of this research.

Ethical approval: Ethical approval was obtained from the respected institution where the study was held (no. 038/2019/1806-2/504). Before distributing the questionnaire, nursing students were informed about the study's purposes, anonymity, confidentiality, and voluntary participation. Their completion and return of the questionnaires were treated as implied consent. Completed surveys were stored securely, and password-protected computer data was accessible only to researchers.

References

[1] Dobrowolska B, Palese A. The caring concept, its behaviours and obstacles: Perceptions from a qualitative study of undergraduate nursing students. Nurs Inq, 2016, 23(4), 305–314.

[2] Gillespie H, Kelly M, Duggan S, Dornan T. How do patients experience caring? Scoping review. Patient Educ Couns, 2017, 100(9), 1622–1633.

[3] Khademian Z, Vizeshfar F. Nursing students' perceptions of the importance of caring behaviors. J Adv Nurs, 2008, 61(4), 456–462.

[4] Kursun S, Arslan FT. Nursing students' perceptions of caring in Turkey. HealthMED, 2012, 6(9), 3145–3151.

[5] Labrague LJ, McEnroe-Petitte DM, Papathanasiou IV, Edet OB, Arulappan J, Tsaras K. Nursing students' perceptions of their own caring behaviors: A multicountry study. Int J Nurs Knowl, 2017, 28(4), 225–232.

[6] Lea A, Watson R, Deary IJ. Caring in nursing: A multivariate analysis. J Adv Nurs, 1998, 28(3), 662–671.

[7] Murphy F, Jones S, Edwards M, James J, Mayer A. The impact of nurse education on the caring behaviours of nursing students. Nurse Educ Today, 2009 Feb 1, 29(2), 254–264.

[8] Ray MA, Turkel MC. Caring as emancipatory nursing praxis: The theory of relational-caring complexity. In: A handbook for caring science. Springer Publishing Company, 2018.

[9] Pajnkihar M, McKenna HP, Štiglic G, Vrbnjak D. Fit for practice: Analysis and evaluation of Watson's Theory of Human Caring. Nurs Sci Q, 2017, 30(3), 243–252.

[10] Parker ME, Smith MC. Nursing theories and nursing practice. 4th ed. Philadelphia, F.A. Davis Company, 2015, 500.

[11] Duffy JR. Theories focused on caring. In: Butts JB, Rich KL, Eds. Philosophies and theories for advanced nursing practice. Jones & Bartlett Learning, 2011, 507–523.

[12] Ray MA, Turkel MC. Caring as emancipatory nursing praxis: The theory of relational-caring complexity. In: A handbook for caring science. Springer Publishing Company, 2018.

[13] Labrague LJ, McEnroe-Petitte DM, Papathanasiou IV, Edet OB, Arulappan J, Tsaras K. Nursing students' perceptions of their own caring behaviors: A multicountry study. Int J Nurs Knowl, 2017, 28(4), 225–232.

[14] Duffy JR. Theories focused on caring. In: Butts JB, Rich KL, Eds. Philosophies and theories for advanced nursing practice. Jones & Bartlett Learning, 2011, 507–523.

[15] Glenn LA, Stocker-Schnieder J, McCune R, McClelland M, King D. Caring nurse practice in the intrapartum setting: Nurses' perspectives on complexity, relationships and safety. J Adv Nurs, 2014 Sep, 70(9), 2019–2030.

[16] Vrbnjak D. Caring for patient and safety in medication administration in nursing: Doctoral thesis. University of Maribor; 2017.

[17] Pajnkihar M, Kocbek P, Musović K, Tao Y, Kasimovskaya N, Štiglic G, et al. An international cross-cultural study of nursing students' perceptions of caring. Nurse Educ Today, 2020, 84, 1–7.

[18] Begum S, Slavin H. Perceptions of "caring" in nursing education by Pakistani nursing students: An exploratory study. Nurse Educ Today, 2012 Apr, 32(3), 332–336.

[19] Labrague LJ, McEnroe-Petitte DM, Papathanasiou IV, Edet OB, Arulappan J, Tsaras K, et al. Nursing students' perceptions of their instructors' caring behaviors: A four-country study. Nurse Educ Today, 2016, 41, 44–49.

[20] Pajnkihar M, Kocbek P, Musović K, Tao Y, Kasimovskaya N, Štiglic G, et al. An international cross-cultural study of nursing students' perceptions of caring. Nurse Educ Today, 2020, 84, 1–7.

[21] Dobrowolska B, Palese A. The caring concept, its behaviours and obstacles: Perceptions from a qualitative study of undergraduate nursing students. Nurs Inq, 2016, 23(4), 305–314.

[22] Karaöz S. Turkish nursing students' perception of caring. Nurse Educ Today, 2005, 25(1), 31–40.

[23] Kursun S, Arslan FT. Nursing students' perceptions of caring in Turkey. HealthMed, 2012, 6(9), 3145–3151.

[24] Wade GH, Kasper N. Nursing students' perceptions of instructor caring: An instrument based on Watson's Theory of Transpersonal Caring. J Nurs Educ, 2006, 45(5), 162–168.

[25] Sanders KM. The impact of immersion on perceived caring in undergraduate nursing students. Int J Caring Sci, 2016, 9(3), 801–809.

[26] Begum S, Slavin H. Perceptions of "caring" in nursing education by Pakistani nursing students: An exploratory study. Nurse Educ Today, 2012 Apr, 32(3), 332–336.

[27] Hills M, Cara C. Curriculum development processes and pedagogical practices for advancing caring science literacy. In: A handbook for caring science. New York, NY, Springer Publishing Company, 2018.

[28] Duffy JR. Learning quality caring. In: Quality caring in nursing and health professions: Implications for clinicians, educators, and leaders. 3rd ed. New York, NY, Springer Publishing Company, 2018, 249–282.

[29] Flack LL, Thrall D. Developing values and philosophies of being. In: A handbook for caring science. New York, NY, Springer Publishing Company, 2018.

[30] Willis DG, Leona-Sheehan DM. Watson's philosophy and theory of transpersonal caring. In: Alligood MR, Ed. Nursing theorists and their work. 9th ed. St. Louis, Elsevier, 2018, 66–79.

[31] Salehian M, Heydari A, Aghebati N, Karimi Moonaghi H, Mazloom SR. Principle-based concept analysis: Caring in nursing education. Electron Physician, 2016 Mar, 8(3), 2160–2167.

[32] Pajnkihar M, McKenna HP, Štiglic G, Vrbnjak D. Fit for practice: Analysis and evaluation of Watson's Theory of Human Caring. Nurs Sci Q, 2017, 30(3), 243–252.

[33] Stanaway JD, Afshin A, Gakidou E, Lim SS, Abate D, Abate KH, et al. Global, regional, and national comparative risk assessment of 84 behavioural, environmental and occupational, and metabolic risks or clusters of risks for 195 countries and territories, 1990–2017:

A systematic analysis for the Global Burden of Disease Stu. Lancet, 2018, 392(10159), 1923–1994.

[34] Labrague LJ. Caring competencies of baccalaureate nursing students of Samar State University. J Nurs Educ Pract, 2012, 2(4), 105–113.

[35] Pajnkihar M, Kocbek P, Musović K, Tao Y, Kasimovskaya N, Štiglic G, et al. An international cross-cultural study of nursing students' perceptions of caring. Nurse Educ Today, 2020, 84, 1–7.

[36] Warshawski S, Itzhaki M, Barnoy S. The associations between peer caring behaviors and social support to nurse students' caring perceptions. Nurse Educ Pract, 2018 Jul, 1(31), 88–94.

[37] Musović K, Štiglic G, Vrbnjak D, Pajnkihar M. Perceptions of caring among Croatian undergraduate nursing students. In: Pajnkihar M, Čuček Trifkovič K, Štiglic G, Eds. Book of Abstracts/International Scientific Conference "Research and Education in Nursing", June 13th 2019, Maribor, Slovenia [Internet]. Maribor, Univerza v Mariboru, Univerzitetna založba, 2019, [cited 2020 Feb 19], 15. Available from: https://plus.si.cobiss.net/opac7/bib/2503332.

[38] Labrague LJ, McEnroe-Petitte DM, Papathanasiou IV, Edet OB, Arulappan J, Tsaras K, et al. Nursing students' perceptions of their instructors' caring behaviors: A four-country study. Nurse Educ Today, 2016, 41, 44–49.

[39] Wade GH, Kasper N. Nursing students' perceptions of instructor caring: An instrument based on Watson's Theory of Transpersonal Caring. J Nurs Educ, 2006, 45(5), 162–168.

[40] Fahey Bacon P. Cultivating caring in nursing education. St. Catherine University, 2012.

[41] Drumm JT. The student's experience of learning caring in a college of nursing grounded in a caring philosophy. [Boca Raton], Florida Atlantic University, 2006.

[42] Sitzman KL, Watson J, Eds. Assessing and measuring caring in nursing and health sciences. 3rd ed. New York, NY, Springer Publishing Company, 2019.

[43] Duffy JR. Learning quality caring. In: Quality caring in nursing and health professions: Implications for clinicians, educators, and leaders. 3rd ed. New York, NY, Springer Publishing Company, 2018, 249–282.

[44] Watson J. Intentionality and caring-healing consciousness. Holist Nurs Pract, 2002, 16(4), 12–19.

[45] Qualtricks. Sample Size Calculator [Internet]. 2022 [cited 2022 Mar 31]. Available from: https://www.qualtrics.com/blog/calculating-sample-size/

[46] Sitzman KL, Watson J, Eds. Assessing and measuring caring in nursing and health sciences. 3rd ed. New York, NY, Springer Publishing Company, 2019.

[47] Polit DF, Beck CT. Nursing research: Generating and assessing evidence for nursing practice. 9th ed. Philadelphia, Wolters Kluwer, 2020.

[48] Johnson VE. Revised standards for statistical evidence. Proc Natl Acad Sci U S A, 2013 Nov 26, 110(48), 19313–19317.

[49] Jönsson P, Wohlin C. An evaluation of k-nearest neighbour imputation using Likert data. In: Proceedings of the 10th International Symposium on Software Metrics. Chicago: IEEE, 2004, 108–118.

[50] R Core Team R. A language and environment for statistical computing. Vienna, Austria, R Foundation for Statistical Computing, 2021.

[51] Mlinar S. First- and third-year student nurses' perceptions of caring behaviours. Nurs Ethics, 2010, 17(4), 491–500.

[52] Bagnall LA, Taliaferro D, Underdahl L. Nursing students, caring attributes, and opportunities for educators. Int J Hum Caring, 2018, 22(3), 126–135.

[53] Murphy F, Jones S, Edwards M, James J, Mayer A. The impact of nurse education on the caring behaviours of nursing students. Nurse Educ Today, 2009 Feb 1, 29(2), 254–264.

[54] Karaöz S. Turkish nursing students' perception of caring. Nurse Educ Today, 2005, 25(1), 31–40.

[55] Pajnkihar M, McKenna HP, Štiglic G, Vrbnjak D. Fit for practice: Analysis and evaluation of Watson's theory of human caring. Nurs Sci Q, 2017, 30(3), 243–252.

[56] Henderson D, Sewell KA, Wei H. The impacts of faculty caring on nursing students' intent to graduate: A systematic literature review. Int J Nurs Sci, 2020, 7(1), 105–111.

[57] Zajac L, Lanem Adrianne J. Student perceptions of faculty presence and caring in accelerated online courses. Q Rev Distance Educ, 2021, 21(2), 67–78.

[58] Jones K, Raynor P, Polyakova-Norwood V. Faculty caring behaviors in online nursing education: An integrative review. 2020.

[59] Jones K, Polyakova-Norwood V, Raynor P, Tavakoli A. Student perceptions of faculty caring in online nursing education: A mixed-methods study. Nurse Educ Today, 2022, 112(March), 105328.

[60] Jones K, Polyakova-Norwood V, Raynor P, Tavakoli A. Student perceptions of faculty caring in online nursing education: A mixed-methods study. Nurse Educ Today, 2022, 112(March), 105328.

[61] Chant S, Jenkinson T, Randale J, Russell G. Communication skills: Some problems in nursing education and practice. J Clin Nurs, 2002, 11.

[62] Sword R. Communication in the Classroom | Skills for Teachers [Internet]. 2020 [cited 2022 Apr 5]. Available from: https://www.highspeedtraining.co.uk/hub/communication-skills-for-teachers/

[63] Torregosa MB, Ynalvez MA, Morin KH. Perceptions matter: Faculty caring, campus racial climate and academic performance. J Adv Nurs, 2016, 72(4), 864–877.

Leona Cilar Budler, Marija Spevan, Kasandra Musović,
Margaret Denny, Suzanne Denieffe, Gregor Štiglic,
Klavdija Čuček Trifkovič

14 Young people's decision to study nursing

Abstract

Introduction: Choosing a career is an extremely important decision for an individual. It is usually based on parental guidance, the decision and influence of friends, or personal desire. Often the motivation to study decreases over the years of study and consequently decreases academic success and satisfaction with the study. Therefore, it is essential to determine which factors affect student motivation.

Methods: We conducted a cross-sectional study among nursing students in Croatia and Slovenia in 2019. A questionnaire on the motivation of nursing students to study was used to collect the data. We used the R statistical software for data analyses.

Results: In total, 312 undergraduate nursing students completed the survey. The sample consisted of 233 (74.7%) participants from Slovenia and 79 (25.2%) from Croatia. Students who feel that studying takes up a lot of their time and affects their social life are less motivated to study.

Discussion: In general, study motivation is related to one's interests in the programme, goals, and wishes. Also, students with a higher level of study motivation are more successful in studying.

Conclusion: It is important to focus research on activities motivating students to choose nursing, maintaining interest and will to study, and activities focused on enhancing student satisfaction with the study. Due to the current shortage in the nursing profession, we should facilitate the motivation of students to pursue a degree already in high school.

Keywords: Nursing, motivation, education

14.1 Introduction

Nursing students' academic motivation is a broad and multidimensional concept influenced by various personal, family, social, educational, and professional factors. It is considered an important factor in academic success, satisfaction, anxiety reduction, continuing education, better learning, creativity, and skill acquisition in nursing [1]. Career choice is an individual's selection of a vocation. It is usually based on parental guidance, an individual's motivation to study, and individual's preferences. People with good career motivation show positive attitudes towards their chosen career and career adaptability and are more optimistic about their future [2]. Mäenpää et al. [3, 4] stated that the key factor for a successful study is the motivation to learn. Students with higher motivation to learn are less likely to experience work burnout [5]. Thus, the students must enter their chosen study with a high level of motivation so that the level of motivation does not decrease.

Students with a higher level of study motivation are more successful, meaning that they achieve better study results. Wu's [6] research findings show that positive academic motivation is important for students to achieve greater academic engagement and achievement, which significantly affects students. Academic success is often influenced by student motivation regulation, study engagement, and experienced burnout regardless of the learning environment [4]. Young people perceive nursing as a career with limited autonomy, shift work, and poor working conditions. The factors influencing the young people's perception are often family and relatives, friends, media, significant others, and other personal factors [7]. Family is a powerful factor that influences students' career choice in nursing [8]. Also, family support, as well as friends' support, has a significant impact on student motivation, stressors, and the intent to leave the study [9].

It is known that nursing students often lose their motivation during their studies. Saeedi and Parvizy [10] found that few strategies could be implemented to improve academic motivation in nursing students. Strategies are directed to professors, students, clinical education, and faculty. It was shown that professors empowering and motivating students towards creating positive attitudes towards nursing, and encouraging academic achievement were assessed as effective strategies in improving students' motivation. On the other hand, novel strategies that also have the potential to motivate nursing students are available. Li et al. [11] examined the efficacy of mobile learning on satisfaction and motivation. The authors found that students showed better study performance after practising mobile learning.

It is important to assess reasons influencing student motivation to develop, evaluate, and implement activities to increase student motivation and, consequently, student's academic achievements and study satisfaction.

14.2 Methods

14.2.1 Study design

We conducted a cross-sectional study in 2019 with nursing students in Croatia and Slovenia to investigate why young people decide to enter the nursing study.

14.2.2 Participants

The study was conducted among 312 undergraduate nursing students in Croatia and Slovenia: 233 from Slovenia and 79 from Croatia. A convenience sampling method was used to include a large number of students in both groups. The following eligibility criteria were used: students studying "general nursing" program, full-time or part-time students, and students in their first, second, or third year of study. Students enrolled in master's or doctoral degree programmes were excluded from this study due to the study aim. With a total number of 625 students, the sample size was calculated using the Raosoft sample size calculator (Raosoft Inc.) using the 5% margin of error, 95% confidence level, and 50% response distribution which resulted in 239 minimum recommended size of the sample.

14.2.3 Setting

Questionnaires were distributed by the researchers online to the Croatian students and in-person prior to the lectures to the Slovenian students between April and June 2019.

14.2.4 Measures

To collect the data, we developed and validated the motivation to study nursing questionnaire [12]. The questionnaire consisted of demographic questions (e.g., gender, faculty, year of study, and employment status) and items on the nursing students' motivation (NSM) scale. The NSM scale included questions about factors to study nursing, general student motivation, general academic success, advantages and disadvantages, reasons to study nursing, and satisfaction with nursing. The response range was 1–5, where 1 represents "I completely disagree" and 5 represents "I completely agree". Questions on the advantages and disadvantages of studying nursing were open [12].

14.2.5 Data analyses

Collected data were analysed using R statistical software version 4.1.0 [13]. Descriptive and statistical methods were used to describe sample characteristics and to check for correlations. We used the R package corrplot [14] to visualize the correlation matrix. There were no missing data.

14.3 Results

14.3.1 Descriptive characteristics of the sample

Three hundred and twelve undergraduate nursing students fulfilled questionnaires and agreed to participate in the study: 233 (74.7%) were from Slovenia and 79 (25.2%) from Croatia. There were 256 (82.1%) female and 56 (17.9%) male participants. Most of the students (n = 218, 69.4%) studied full time.

14.3.2 Student motivation

Students were asked to evaluate their general motivation on a scale from 1 to 5, where 1 meant entirely unmotivated, and 5 meant entirely motivated. The mean value for motivation was 14.28 (SD = 2.61), with a minimum score of 5 and a maximum of 21.

14.3.3 Influences of various factors on motivation to study

Participants were asked about persons who influenced their decision to enter nursing studies. About 78.3% (n = 246) participants stated that no other person influenced on their decision, 11.1% (n = 35) stated that parents had influence, and 4.5% (n = 14) stated that friends had influence. Moreover, student motivation was assessed using the following items: thinking about quitting study if having bad grades, thinking about other study programmes, choosing nursing even if the nursing study would influence social life, thinking about quitting study if studying took more than 60 h per week, and regretting if did not choose nursing as a study program. The data distribution of items is shown in Fig. 14.1.

In Fig. 14.2, the data distribution of each scale component is presented.

The correlation between various factors (gender, high school, and influence) and motivation to study is presented in Fig. 14.3. A positive correlation is marked with blue and a negative correlation with red. An insignificant correlation is not marked with colour.

Student motivation is higher in students who were sure they wanted to study nursing and did not consider entering other studies (r = 0.68). Also, the correlation is strongly positive between student motivation and items describing that they would regret if they did not choose nursing as a study program (r = 0.61). There is a correlation between student motivation and study influence on social life (r = 0.62). Students with many obligations are less successful in their studies (r = −0.32).

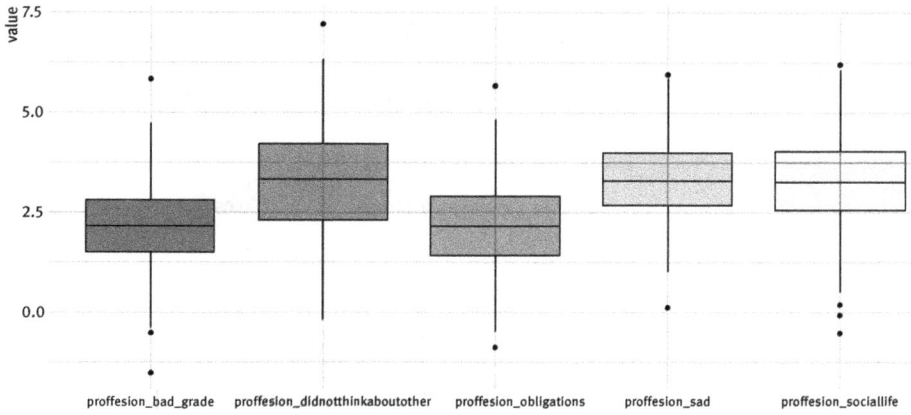

Fig. 14.1: Data distribution among student motivation items.

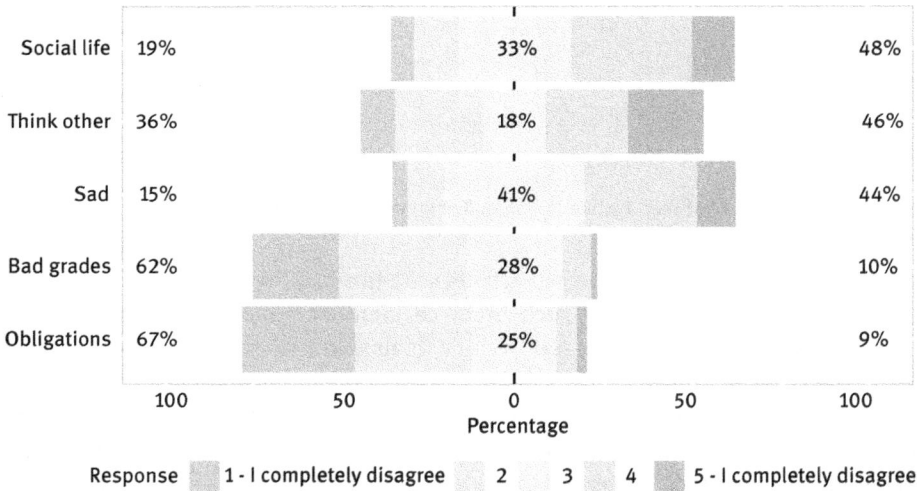

Fig. 14.2: Likert-scale response distribution for student motivation items.

14.4 Discussion

This study aimed to determine which factors influence students' motivation to choose a nursing degree programme. Career planning is a demanding process where every decision has its consequences. Students' skills and intentions may change completely depending on the type and specific career choice [15]. The motivation of the students who participated in this study is slightly higher than average. Motivation included processes

	motivation_total	general_motivation	proffesion_sad	proffesion_sociallife	gender	faculty	study_type	study_year	high_school	influence	proffesion_bad_grades	proffesion_obligations
Proffesion_didnotthinkaboutother	0.68	0.19	0.35	0.35	-0.06	0.06	0.14	-0.04	-0.2	0.1	-0.07	-0.17
motivation_total		0.26	0.61	0.62	-0.03	0.01	0.04	0	-0.09	0.05	0.27	0.11
general_motivation			0.45	0.4	0.01	0.02	0.03	0.24	0.09	0.02	-0.13	-0.3
proffesion_sad				0.62	0.03	-0.01	0.03	0.09	0.05	-0.03	-0.16	-0.32
proffesion_sociallife					0.01	-0.05	0.03	0.08	0.01	0.05	-0.21	-0.29
gender						0.04	0.09	0.04	0.01	-0.05	0	0.03
faculty							0.49	0.05	-0.21	-0.07	-0.05	-0.02
study_type								0.1	-0.15	0.14	-0.13	-0.02
study_year									0.06	-0.04	-0.1	-0.01
high_school										-0.06	0.05	-0.04
influence											-0.02	0.01
proffesion_bad_grades												0.24

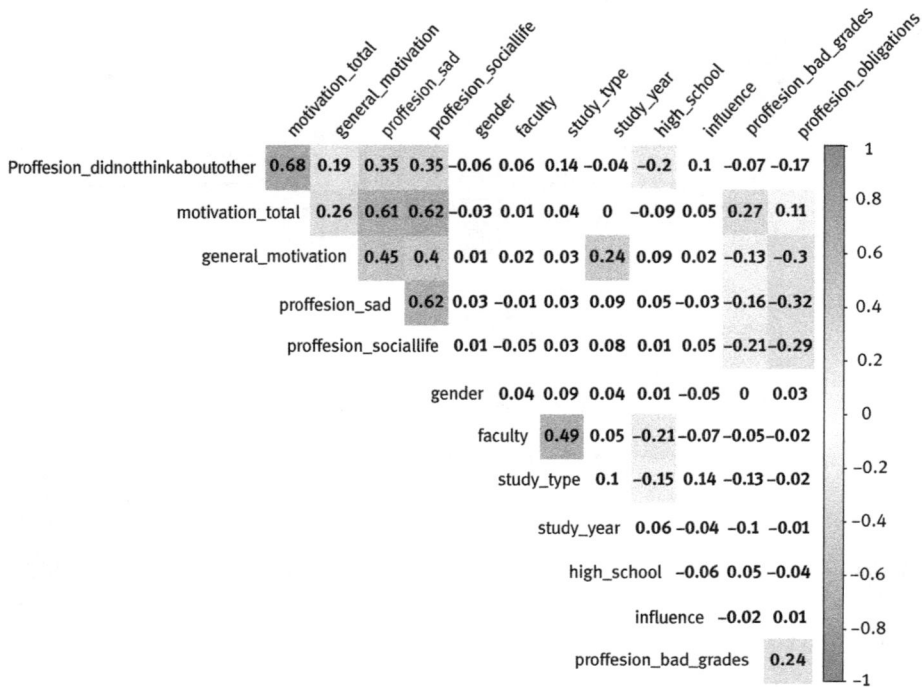

Fig. 14.3: Correlations between motivation to study nursing and various factors.

to promote and sustain goal-directed activities. Motivational processes can be internal influences that lead to outcomes such as choice, effort, persistence, or success. Important internal motivational processes include goals and self-evaluations of progress, self-efficacy, social comparisons, values, expectations of outcomes, attribution, and self-regulation [16]. The largest number of students indicates that no one influenced their decision to enrol in nursing, while a smaller number of respondents indicate that their parents and friends influenced them; high parental expectations are positively associated with adolescents' academic success and depression. Complex parental expectations and a mediating role can be very detrimental for young students [17]. Students convinced of their decision to study nursing were more motivated and did not regret choosing this course. Self-efficacy belief is a motivational product. When students can manage their problems and choices, their self-efficacy increases, and they become more motivated to achieve academic success [18]. Motivation is lower in students where education and many commitments interfere with social life or the other way around. Student life balance is an important predictor of student mental health. Educational institutions should emphasize helping students find a balance between student life and personal life so that students can improve their faculty experience [19], and too much workload can lead to dropping out of studies. Motivation is higher among students who did not think about other study programmes or vice versa. Nursing programmes are becoming increasingly popular in many countries [20]. One major reason for choosing nursing is that people want a secure, stable, and respected career with various opportunities [21]. In the same way, motivation is higher among students who would regret that they did not choose nursing as a study programme or inversely.

Motivation is also higher among students who would choose nursing, even if the study would influence their social life or vice versa. A study aimed to determine the prevalence of sleep disorders among nursing students found that chronic sleep deprivation is indirectly responsible for decreased social life in nursing students [22]. However, a high workload and lack of time for social life remain factors in nurses' turnover [23]. However, students who believe that nursing study would affect their social life would still choose to study and would regret it if they did not choose or inversely. The other variables were not as strongly correlated.

However, our study has some limitations regarding study design, sample, and sampling method. Our study was cross-sectional, so it reflects phenomena at a single time point. A longitudinal design might be necessary to explore the phenomena over an extended period and possible changes over time. Another limitation regards our convenience sampling method as it may not represent the typical population, for example, in our sample, 80% of the participants were female, and the results cannot be generalized. In further studies, this might be improved by using a more complex sampling method, such as random stratified sampling. Furthermore, recall bias could also be present, as the higher year students were asked to answer questions about the things from their past. In addition, the disproportion of sample size could have influenced statistical testing.

14.5 Conclusion

In Slovenia, Croatia, and the rest of the world, there is a large shortage of healthcare personnel, which can consequently affect the quality of patient care. Students must recognize the significance of nursing. Furthermore, they must develop a positive attitude towards their profession. Despite various factors that may reduce students' motivation to study, we want them to maintain their highest possible motivation with different support methods and to remain in the nursing profession after graduating.

References

[1] Rafii F, Saeedi M, Parvizy S. Academic motivation in nursing students: A hybrid concept analysis. Iran J Nurs Midwifery Res, 2019, 24(5), 315.

[2] Fang W, Zhang Y, Mei J, Chai X, Fan X. Relationships between optimism, educational environment, career adaptability and career motivation in nursing undergraduates: A cross-sectional study. Nurse Educ Today, 2018, 68, 33–39.

[3] Mäenpää K, Järvenoja H, Peltonen J, Pyhältö K. Progress of nursing students' motivation regulation profiles and affiliations with engagement, burnout and academic performance. Int J Teach Learn Higher Educ, 2019.

[4] Mäenpää K, Järvenoja H, Peltonen J, Pyhältö K. Nursing students' motivation regulation strategies in blended learning: A qualitative study. Nurs Health Sci, 2020, 22(3), 602–611.

[5] Boekaerts M. Engagement as an inherent aspect of the learning process. Learn Instr, 2016, 43, 76–83.

[6] Wu Z. Academic motivation, engagement, and achievement among college students. Coll Stud J, 2019, 53(1), 99–112.

[7] Glerean N, Hupli M, Talman K, Haavisto E. Young peoples' perceptions of the nursing profession: An integrative review. Nurse Educ Today, 2017, 5, 95–102.

[8] Maor S, Cojocaru S. Family as a powerful factor that influences career choice in nursing. Soc Res Rep, 2018, 10(1).

[9] Volkert D, Candela L, Bernacki M. Student motivation, stressors, and intent to leave nursing doctoral study: A national study using path analysis. Nurse Educ Today, 2018, 61, 210–215.

[10] Saeedi M, Parvizy S. Strategies to promote academic motivation in nursing students: A qualitative study. J Educ Health Promot, 2019, 8.

[11] Li KC, Lee LYK, Wong SL, Yau ISY, Wong BTM. Effects of mobile apps for nursing students: Learning motivation, social interaction and study performance. Open Learn J Open Distance e-Learn, 2018, 33(2), 99–114.

[12] Cilar L, Spevan M, Trifkovič KČ, Štiglic G. What motivates students to enter nursing? Findings from a cross-sectional study. Nurse Educ Today, 2020, 90, 104463.

[13] R Core Team: A language and environment for statistical computing. R Foundation for Statistical Computing, Vienna, Austria. 2017. Accessed from: https://www.Rproject.org/.

[14] Wei T, Simko V, Levy M, Xie Y, Jin Y, Zemla J. Package' corrplot'. Statistician, 2017, 56(316), e24.

[15] Hutchison B, Niles SG. Career development theories. In: Stebnicki MA, Marini I, eds. The professional counselor's desk reference. 2nd ed. New York, NY, USA, Springer Publishing Company, 2016, 285–289.

[16] Schunk DH, DiBenedetto MK. Motivation and social cognitive theory. Contemp Educ Psychol, 2020, 60, 101832.

[17] Ma Y, Siu A, Tse WS. The role of high parental expectations in adolescents' academic performance and depression in Hong Kong. J Fam Issues, 2018, 39(9), 2505–2522.

[18] Bernacki ML, Nokes-Malach TJ, Aleven V. Examining self-efficacy during learning: Variability and relations to behavior, performance, and learning. Metacogn Learn, 2015, 10(1), 99–117.

[19] Sprung JM, Rogers A. Work-life balance as a predictor of college student anxiety and depression. J Am Coll Health, 2020, 69(7), 1–8.

[20] Mckenna L, Brooks I. Graduate entry student's early perceptions on their future nursing careers. Nurse Educ Pract, 2018, 28(1), 292–295.

[21] Wilkes L, Cowin L, Johnson M. The reasons students choose to undertake a nursing degree. Collegian, 2015, 22(3), 259–265.

[22] Guabfredi V, Nucci D, Tonzani A, Amodeo R, Benvenuti AL, Millarini M, et al. Sleep disorder, mediterranean diet and learning performance among nursing students: Insomnia, a cross-sectional study. 2018, 30(6), 470–481.

[23] Holland P, Leng Tham T, Sheehan C, Cooper B. The impact of perceived workload on nurse satisfaction with work-life balance and intention to leave the occupation. Appl Nurs Res, 2019, 49(2019), 70–76.

Gregor Štiglic, Leona Cilar Budler, Roger Watson

15 Running a confirmatory factor analysis in R: a step-by-step tutorial

Abstract

Introduction: Confirmatory factor analysis is a frequently used data analysis technique in nursing research for the development of new measures and psychometric evaluation. R is an open-source statistical software for data analysis that allows a high level of reproducibility required for submission in more and more scientific journals in nursing. The aim of this chapter is to provide a step-by-step tutorial for conducting confirmatory factor analysis in the statistical program R.

Methods: Data collected from 938 students in Scotland who completed the Trait Emotional Intelligence Questionnaire Short form (TEIQue-SF) were used to conduct analyses.

Results: We demonstrated a reproducible way of conducting a correlation-based network visualization followed by confirmatory factor analysis to confirm the four-factor structure in the TEIQue-SF questionnaire.

Conclusion: This chapter focuses on the demonstration of an alternative statistical tool to the frequently used point-and-click software by providing detailed instructions in the form of reproducible code and data.

Keywords: nurses, nursing, R, data analysis, factor analysis, confirmatory factor analysis

15.1 Introduction

R is an open-source, crowd-funded, programming language for statistical computing and graphics [1]. R uses different packages for conducting various functions and analyses. The packages are created by statisticians across the world. Packages are available under a Creative Commons License and are regularly updated and rigorously tested before being made available via CRAN (The Comprehensive R Archive Network) [2, 3]. R can be used with various platforms including Linux, Mac, and Windows [4]. At the time of writing, version 4.0.2 (Taking Off Again) is available. R is not easy to use; it has a "steep learning curve" and can be hard for someone without computer programming experience. On the other hand, it is free (*caveat emptor* applies), and a lot of help is available online. The use of R can be facilitated by installing RStudio® (the basic package is free) and allows the user to store coding. Even with this facility, users must workaround obscure error messages which appear frequently. Although R is a free, powerful, and flexible alternative, it is less familiar and less frequently used in nursing research [5].

Healthcare institutions must be prepared to invest in new, effective, and efficient treatments and interventions for patient benefit. Before the implementation of new interventions, research must be done using valid and reliable measurements [6]. Questionnaires used for the data collection need to be tested for reliability and validity. When developing and validating the questionnaire, psychometric tests must be conducted. These include, for example, parametric item response theory, factor analysis (FA), and reliability via classical test theory.

Exploratory analysis of data can be conducted to observe the correlations between items as an initial step to statistically more rigorous approaches. Correlation or covariance matrices are usually the simplest techniques that can be used in this step. While such an approach allows good visualization of multiple pairwise correlations, it is unable to capture the more complex correlations among multiple items. One of the novel approaches used in this field is correlation networks that aim, simultaneously, to capture the correlation and grouping of the items in the same visualization and were used in other fields like bioinformatics earlier [7]. However, the technique recently developed in multiple variants of psychological network visualization as a psychometric approach [8].

FA is a method for testing whether item covariance structure justifies the use of item scores to calculate (sub)scale scores [9]. The aim of FA is to reduce "the dimensionality of the original space and to give an interpretation to the new space, spanned by a reduced number of new dimensions which are supposed to underlie the old ones" [10]. Matsunaga [11] discusses the importance of FA and how it is often misunderstood. Although an increasing number of researchers are using these methods, evidence suggests that a large proportion of the research published still harbours ill-informed practices. Thus, it is important that researchers are aware of different FA methods. Confirmatory FA (CFA) is often used for developing a new measure, testing measurement invariance, construct validation, testing method effects, and psychometric evaluation. CFA is strongly related to exploratory FA (EFA), principal component analysis, and structural equation modelling (SEM) [12]. EFA is described as the orderly simplification of interrelated measures. It has been traditionally used to explore the possible underlying factor structure of a set of observed variables without imposing a preconceived structure on the outcome [13]. The result of performing EFA is identification of the underlying factor structure. On the other hand, CFA is used to verify the factor structure of a set of observed variables. It allows testing a relationship between observed variables and the existence of their underlying latent constructs. The researcher can use theoretical knowledge, empirical research, or both; can postulate the relationship pattern a priori; and can then test the hypothesis statistically [14]. Both the EFA and CFA are types of factor analyses based on the common factor model, which proposes that each observed response is influenced partially by the underlying common factors and partially by the underlying unique factors [15]. For conducting CFA, researchers must have strong empirical or conceptual knowledge to guide factor model specification and evaluation [12]. CFA will be described in detail in the following sections.

In this tutorial, we introduce a short step-by-step tutorial on how to perform CFA for researchers using statistics and R programming in applied healthcare research. The corresponding R Markdown script is available as a supplementary material.

15.2 Methods

15.2.1 Design

This chapter represents a tutorial on using the R statistical software to perform CFA and the corresponding exploratory analysis.

15.2.2 Participants

We used the dataset originally from the study by Snowden et al. [16] to examine the construct validity of the Trait Emotional Intelligence Questionnaire Short form (TEIQue-SF). The TEIQue-SF is a short-form questionnaire which includes 30 items. It was developed by Petrides [17] to measure global trait emotional intelligence (trait EI). Petrides derived it from the larger 130-item-based TEIQue questionnaire by Freudenthaler et al. [18]. Items were selected based on their correlations with the corresponding total facet scores [19]. Responses to the TEIQue-SF items are made on a Likert-type scale (e.g., 1 meaning "strongly disagree" and 7 meaning "strongly agree"). The total scale score is derived by summing the score of each item (after reverse scoring of negative items) and is used to locate respondents on the latent trait continuum. A higher score represents a greater presence of the trait EI [20]. Four dimensions of trait EI are measured with the TEIQue-SF: well-being, sociability, self-control, and emotionality. Petrides [17] defines well-being as related feelings of a time based around achievements, self-regard, and expectations; self-control as regulating and having control over emotions, impulses, and stress; emotionality as an ability to perceive, express, and connect with emotions in self and others, which can be used in creating successful interpersonal relationships; and sociability as being socially assertive and aware, managing others' emotions, and effectiveness in communication and participation in social situations. Sample characteristics are presented in Tab. 15.1 [16].

Tab. 15.1: Sample characteristics.

	Programme	Frequency	Per cent	Valid per cent	Cumulative per cent
Valid	Adult	586	62.5	62.5	62.5
	Mental health	124	13.2	13.2	75.8
	Learning disability	29	3.1	3.1	78.9
	Children	47	5.0	5.0	83.9
	Midwifery	83	8.8	8.9	92.7
	Computing	68	7.2	7.3	100.0
	Total	937	99.9	100.0	
Missing	System	1	0.1		
Total		938	100.0		

15.2.3 Data collection

Data were collected from 938 students of nursing, midwifery, and computer science in two Scottish universities. The dataset also contains information on the gender of the participants. The data and R source code are available at the Mendeley Data repository [21].

15.2.4 Data analysis

FA is a common method used to find a small set of unobserved variables (called latent variables, or factors) which can account for the covariance among a set of observed variables (called manifest variables) [22]. Latent variables are variables that are inferred, not directly observed, from other variables that are observed. The presence of latent variables can be detected by their effects on variables that are observable [23]. A manifest variable is a variable or factor that can be directly measured or observed. Commonly, CFA models are displayed as path diagrams in which squares represent observed variables and circles represent the latent concepts. Moreover, single-headed arrows are used to imply a direction of assumed causal influence, and double-headed arrows represent covariance between two latent variables [22].

Initially, we should justify the sample size which allows a robust enough CFA. Determining the appropriate sample size for CFA is a complex task; therefore, we refer the interested readers to read more on this topic in a paper by Kyriazos [24].

Also, before any FA, it is important to test the dataset for FA suitability. There are two methods for testing FA suitability: the Bartlett's Test of Sphericity and the Kaiser, Meyer, Olkin (KMO) test. Those tests are used to check whether a matrix is significantly different from an identity matrix. A significant Bartlett's test of sphericity states that FA may proceed if $p < 0.001$. In 1970, this method was modified by Kaiser as the Measure of Sampling Adequacy (MSA), and in 1974 by Kaiser and Rice [25]. The KMO statistic can vary from 0 to 1 and indicates the degree to which each variable in a set is predicted without error by the other variables. The KMO statistic indicates how much variance in your variables might be caused by underlying factors. High values, close to 1.0, indicate that a factor analysis may be appropriate for your data. CFA is based on the covariances among variances. These are susceptible to the effects of violations to the assumption of normality which can affect covariances. CFA models contain the parameters of factor variances and covariances (Ψ – psi), factor loadings (Λ – lambda), and error factor variances and covariances (Θε – theta–epsilon) [26].

Before running a model, the variables should be examined to check that there are no deviations from normality. The MVN package [27] provides various approaches to check for univariate or multivariate deviation from a normal distribution. In practice, there are many cases where normality will not be met, especially in surveys using Likert scales. In such cases, we can use a robust estimator as presented in Finney and DiStefano [28]. In this tutorial, we used maximum likelihood estimation with robust standard errors and a Satorra–Bentler scaled test statistic which can be used even in cases of deviations from the normality in most or all variables.

A simple exploratory visualization of the data can be performed to check for the correlations between the variables and to see the grouping of the variables in factors. It should be noted that correlation matrices produce different results from CFA when the relationships between the items are observed. Instead of using a correlation matrix, CFA uses a variance–covariance matrix on raw data to estimate input variance [12]. In this chapter, we present an example of correlation visualization using correlation network graphs [29]. Correlation graphs have been used to visualize relations and the grouping of variables at the same time. However, the most frequently used force-directed positioning of the network nodes representing variables is not easily interpretable and can be misleading when grouping of the variables is observed. Therefore, alternative options are available in the qgraph package [29]. In this chapter, we used multidimensional scaling to position nodes resulting in a more realistic grouping of nodes [8].

First, the factor loadings of the indicators (observed variables) that make up the latent construct need to be calculated. The standardized factor loading squared is the estimate of the amount of the variance of the indicator that is accounted for by the latent construct. Factor loadings of 0.4 or higher are acceptable [30]. The unique variance is not explained by the latent construct. We also need to check the convergent validity of the construct, which is indicated by high indicator loadings, which shows the strength of how well the indicators are theoretically similar. Most models contain more than one factor. In that case, we need to run a CFA for all the model's latent constructs within one measurement model. Discriminant validity exists when no two constructs are highly correlated. If two constructs are highly correlated (> 0.85), we need to explore combining the constructs.

Many different approaches are proposed to assess the fit of the model to the data [31]. Some of the more popular fit statistics include the comparative fit index (CFI), the Tucker–Lewis index (TLI), and root mean square error of approximation (RMSEA). CFI is frequently used as it is known to perform well even when the sample size is small [32] and assumes that all latent variables are uncorrelated and compares the postulated model to the null model. The CFI values can range from 0.0 to 1.0, where values close to 1.0 represent a good fit. To avoid misspecified models it is generally advised for models to achieve CFI over 0.90 which represents a good fit with some authors arguing that the threshold should lie at 0.95 [33]. TLI measures a relative reduction in misfit per degree of freedom [34] with threshold values of 0.90 indicating adequate fit and 0.95 indicating good fit [35]. On the other hand, the RMSEA represents a so-called badness-of-fit measure resulting in lower values for a better fit. It measures discrepancy due to the approximation with values below 0.06 representing an acceptable model [36].

15.3 Results

In this section, we provide step-by-step instructions on how to run the CFA analysis.

15.3.1 Step 1: reading and checking the data

In the initial step, we read the data from the CSV file using the read.csv command in R. After reading the data, we checked whether the data were loaded by using a command str which prints the summary information on the structure of the data just loaded. This way it is possible to print the type and a few example values for each variable. In the case of the TEIQue-SF example data provided with this chapter, we observe that our data consists of 938 samples with 36 variables. It needs to be noted that as in most real-world datasets only a specific number of variables will be used in the CFA analysis. In our case, only 30 variables are TEIQue-SF scale variables. Items from the TEIQue-SF scale will be used in the CFA analysis. As mentioned, it is important that the researcher who is performing a CFA has knowledge about the scale and its basic properties. Thus, we removed items 3, 18, 14, and 29 that were considered as a "general" factor by Petrides and Furnham [19], and we were left with 26 items that should represent 4 factors: well-being, self-control, emotionality, and sociability. For visualization needed in the next step, we also import textual description for each item containing the questions for all 30 items.

In addition to the above-mentioned data reading and checking functions, the following packages need to be loaded in R: smacof (multidimensional scaling needed for exploratory analysis in our case), parameters (KMO and Bartlet's test), lavaan (CFA analysis), qgraph (visualization for exploratory analysis), and semplot (visualization of the relations between items and factors). The initial steps are shown in Box 15.1.

Box 15.1: Source code for exploratory analysis.

```
library(qgraph)
library(lavaan)
library(semPlot)
library(smacof)
library(parameters)
# Load the data from a csv file
data <- read.csv("db_TEIQ_CFA_SCO.csv", header = T)
# Print some information on the data we just read to check
# whether the data loaded properly
str(data)
# Separate TEIQue-SF values in a variable named teiq
teiq <- data[,2:31]
# Load item names
names <- readLines("items.txt")
# Create variable names for TEIQue-SF data (V1 – V30)
colnames(teiq) <- paste0("V", 1:30)
# Items 3, 18, 14 & 29 were omitted from the CFA because
# Petrides (2006) considered them a 'general' factor as
# they were not specifically associated with any particular factor.
# Additionally, item number 20 was omitted as suggested by
# Snowden et al. (2016)
teiq <- teiq[,-c(3, 18, 14, 29, 20)]
names <- names[-c(3, 18, 14, 29, 20)]
# Rearange columns and related questions to match four subscales
items <- c("V30","V15","V19","V24","V27","V21","V9","V6",
"V12","V5","V28","V13","V16",
"V7","V10","V22","V25","V8","V4","V2",
"V11","V26","V17","V1","V23")
pos <- match(items, colnames(teiq))
teiq <- teiq[,items]
names <- names[pos]
```

15.3.2 Step 2: exploratory data analysis

The Bartlett's test of sphericity and the KMO tests were conducted as shown in Box 15.2 to test if the dataset is suitable for FA. Moreover, variables were examined to check for deviations from normality using univariate (Shapiro–Wilk) and multivariate (Henze–Zirkler) tests of normality.

The KMO MSA suggests that the data are appropriate for FA (KMO = 0.88). Bartlett's test of sphericity suggests that there is sufficient significant correlation in the data for FA ($\chi^2(300) = 4{,}841.03$, $p < 0.001$). On the other hand, none of the items is normally distributed and consequently, the multivariate normality test shows the same. Since we are using Likert-scale items, this is not unusual, but it requires a different approach to the CFA. In our case, a robust estimator following Finney and DiStefano [28] was used to perform CFA on non-normally distributed data. More specifically, we used maximum likelihood estimation with robust standard errors and a Satorra–Bentler scaled test statistic.

Box 15.2: Source code for basic CFA data assessment.

```
# KMO and Bartlet's test
check_factorstructure(teiq)
# Univariate (Shapiro-Wilk) and multivariate (Henze-Zirkler) test of normal distribution
result <- mvn(data = teiq, mvnTest = "hz", univariateTest = "SW", desc = TRUE)
result$univariateNormality
result$multivariateNormality
```

Next, we used a simple exploratory visualization of the data to check the correlations between the variables and potentially already see the grouping of variables into four factors. This can be done using the R command qgraph (Fig. 15.1 and Box 15.3).

Box 15.3: Visualization of the data using correlation graph.

```
# Define a vector of item groups belonging to subscales
groups <- c(rep('Confidence', 8), rep('Connection', 5),
rep('Uncertainty', 7), rep('Empathy', 5))
group_col <- c("#72CF53", "#53B0CF", "#FFB026", "#ED3939")
# Covariance matrix
corMat <- cov(teiq, use = "pairwise.complete.obs")
# Multidimensional scaling based positioning of the nodes in the network
dissimilarity <- sim2diss(cor(teiq))
mdsModel <- mds(dissimilarity)
head(round(mdsModel$conf, 2))
png(filename = "figure2.png", type = "cairo", height = 6, width = 12, units = 'in', res = 300)
qgraph(corMat, graph = "cor", sampleSize = nrow(data),
layout = mdsModel$conf, color = group_col,vsize = 4, esize = 4,
border.width = 2, border.color = "black", groups = groups,
nodeNames = names, legend = TRUE, legend.mode = "style1",
legend.cex = .36, theme = "colorblind",
threshold = "bonferroni",
minimum = "sig", alpha = 0.05)
dev.off()
```

Confidence

- ○ V30: Others admire me for being relaxed.
- ○ V15: On the whole, I'm able to deal with stress.
- ○ V19: I'm able to find ways to control my emotions.
- ○ V24: I believe I'm full of personal strengths.
- ○ V27: I generally believe that things will work out fine in my life.
- ○ V21: I would describe myself as a good negotiator.
- ○ V9: I feel that I have a number of good qualities.
- ○ V6: I can deal effectively with people.

Connection

- ○ V12: On the whole, I have a gloomy perspective on most things.
- ○ V5: I generally don't find life enjoyable.
- ○ V28: I find it difficult to bond well even with those close to me.
- ○ V13: Those close to me often complain that I don't treat them right.
- ○ V16: I find it difficult to show my affection to those close to me.

Empathy

- ○ V11: I'm usually able to influence the way other people feel.
- ○ V26: I don't seem to have any power over other people's feelings.
- ○ V17: I'm able to "get into someone's shoes".
- ○ V1: Expressing my emotions with words is not a problem for me.
- ○ V23: I often pause and think about my feelings.

Uncertainty

- ○ V7: I tend to change my mind frequently.
- ○ V10: I often find it difficult to stand up for my rights.
- ○ V22: I tend to get involved in things I later wish I could get out of.
- ○ V25: I tend to "back down" even if I know I'm right.
- ○ V8: Many times, I can't figure out what emotion I'm feeling.
- ○ V4: I usually find it difficult to regulate my emotions.
- ○ V2: I find it difficult to see things from another person's viewpoint.

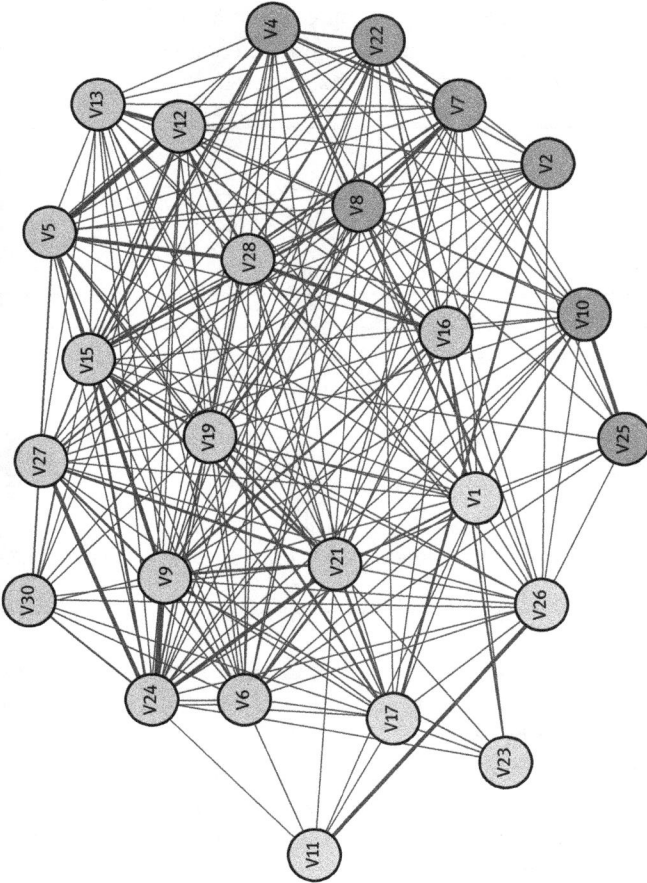

Fig. 15.1: Exploratory analysis of data using correlation graphs.

15.3.3 Step 3: building CFA model

We specified the laavan specific model, where each line represents a single latent factor with its indicators following the = ~ as shown in Box 15.4. In the code, we defined four latent factors referring to trait EI: confidence, connection, uncertainty, and empathy. We are assuming that 25 variables are indicators of those latent factors.

15.3.4 Step 4: examine model fit statistics

In the next step, a model was fitted to the TEIQue-SF data using the command model.fit from the laavan package, and is followed by printing a summary of the CFA results after fitting the model to the data as shown in Box 15.5. The laavan command summary provides a very extensive list of the CFA results with many details. However, most of the users will be interested in some of the basic CFA measures such as CFI, TLI, or RMSEA that can be obtained by a simple command fitMeasures as demonstrated in the supplementary materials in this chapter.

Box 15.4: CFA analysis using laavan package.
model <- 'Confidence = ~ V30 + V15 + V19 + V24 + V27 + V21 + V9 + V6
Connection = ~ V12 + V5 + V28 + V13 + V16
Uncertainty = ~ V7 + V10 + V22 + V25 + V8 + V4 + V2
Empathy = ~ V11 + V26 + V17 + V1 + V23'

Box 15.5: Examination of model fit, including visualization of the model.
model.fit <- cfa(model, teiq, std.lv = TRUE, missing = "fiml")
# Print model summary
summary(model.fit, fit.measures = TRUE, standardized = TRUE)
# Print only selected fit measures
fitMeasures(model.fit, c("cfi","tli", "rmsea"))
# Visualize normalized values for all items and corresponding factors
semPaths(model.fit, what = "std", layout = 'circle2', intercepts = FALSE, residuals = FALSE, nCharNodes = 10)

The fit of our four-factor model resulted in RMSEA = 0.058, CFI = 0.818 (NB: these values are identical to those obtained by Snowden et al. [16]), TLI = 0.797, and SRMR = 0.054 (NB: these values were not reported by Snowden et al.). Although some of the results like CFI or TLI are below the generally accepted threshold of 0.9, point at weak fit, one should be careful when relying on the CFA threshold values. As a final step of the CFA, we used semPaths command from the semPath package in R which can be used to visualize normalized values for all items and corresponding four factors (Fig. 15.2).

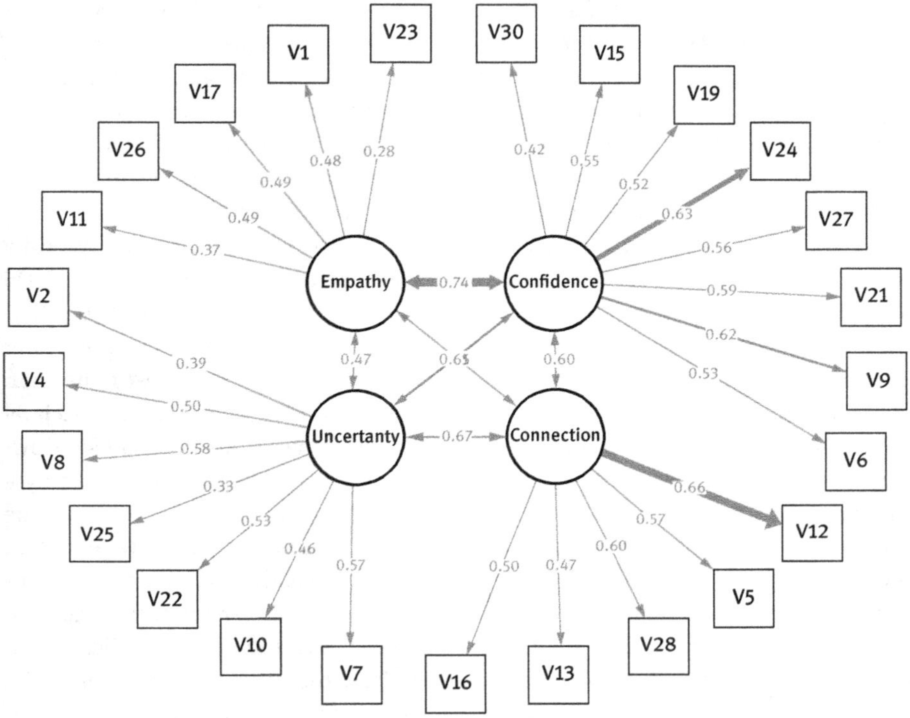

Fig. 15.2: Visualization of the obtained CFA model.

15.4 Discussion

The aim of research in nursing is the delivery of evidence-based care [37]. To collect and analyse the data, researchers need to have sufficient statistics, informatics and programming knowledge, and work experience. There are several software packages available for conducting various statistical analyses, which differ in capabilities for handling single group, multiple groups, non-normal variables, and missing data [38]. Although R is free to use, it is complex to use for clinicians with no statistical educational background. Thus, step-by-step tutorials and available scripts can help new or potential users in the transition from alternative, usually more costly, solutions.

Thus, we set out in this chapter to demonstrate, generally, the use of the R programming language for statistical analysis and, specifically, to demonstrate how to run a CFA using R [39]. Therefore, we were less concerned with establishing the structure of the TEIQue-SF, which had already been established in a previous study, than with demonstrating the utility of the R programming language. In this light, the study was conducted against a background of very few "user-friendly" articles explaining how to use R for a specific analysis and especially to nurses who are not, traditionally, comfortable with the use of statistics [40]. Typical of the genre of articles purporting to introduce the use of R for a specific analysis is a study by Ritz and Striebig [41] in the *Journal of Statistical Software* which assumes considerable prior knowledge of programming generally and R specifically. Books and manuals on using R notoriously suffer from the same problems.

To conduct this study, we used a dataset that had already been analysed by CFA using the commercial package and IBM SPSS "bolt on" IBM programme AMOS (Analysis of Moment Structures) and published by Snowden et al. [16]. The differences between these two packages are striking. AMOS is modestly priced at under USD 100 but requires to be run alongside SPSS for which licenses cost more than USD 1,000. It should be noted that in some cases the price can be lower, especially with a student or campus-wide licensing. On the other hand, R is free to use. However, the facilities in AMOS are relatively much more user-friendly requiring only a minimum of technical skill to run [42]. The most attractive feature of AMOS is the ability to draw the path diagrams and, thereby, to visualize the structural equation models that are being analysed [38]. These can also be easily modified and the outputs – both graphical and numerical – are quite easy to understand, provided the user has a reasonable understanding of SEM, generally, and CFA, specifically. On the other hand, while we demonstrate that precisely the same outcomes for a CFA are obtained using either AMOS or R, the process of using R is considerably less intuitive. Unlike a commercial package such as AMOS – where the output includes all parameters including fit indices and a visual representation of the data – R requires multiple steps and the coordinated use of several different statistical packages. But R does have some additional features over AMOS and that the output of SEM can be easily visualized and in a form that is easily used in presentations and publications. Moreover, AMOS does not implement complex sampling estimation [43].

15.4.1 Limitations

We readily admit that R is not easy to master, and it is also customary for users only to make use of and have expertise in a limited range of the packages and methods available in R. Towards the end of helping other users, we provide in detail and in its entirety the R coding used in the present analysis, demonstrating how to load packages and subsequently to run specific aspects of the analysis. For others wishing to conduct CFA in R, we encourage simply by copying and pasting this coding into R or R Studio and we also make our database available for others to replicate this analysis. By publishing the code and data we also demonstrate that compared with most other alternatives, R offers a high level of reproducibility.

15.5 Conclusion

CFA is a common data-analytic method used in development of new measures and psychometric evaluation in nursing research. Thus, it is important that researchers have basic knowledge for conducting CFA analysis. CFA can be performed in R following basic steps as proposed in this chapter: reading and checking the data, conducting exploratory data analysis, building CFA model, and examining model fit statistics. R is an alternative statistical tool for conducting statistical analyses in nursing. R also ensures reproducible code and data, provides reproducibility of the results, and offers wide variety of visualization options.

References

[1]   R Development Core Team. A language and environment for statistical computing. Vienna, Austria, R Foundation for Statistical Computing, 2005.

[2]   Beaujean AA. Factor analysis using R. Practical Assess Res Eval, 2013, 18(1), 4.

[3]   Venables WN, Smith DM. R development core team. An introduction to R. Vienna, Austria, R Foundation for Statistical Computing, 2009.

[4]   Ozgur C, Kleckner M, Li Y. Selection of statistical software for solving big data problems: A guide for businesses, students, and universities. SAGE Open, 2015, 5(2), 2158244015584379.

[5]   Stiglic G, Watson R, Cilar L. R you ready? Using the R programme for statistical analysis and graphics. Res Nurs Health, 2019, 42(6), 494–499.

[6]   Saha E, Ray PK. Statistical analysis of medical data for inventory management in a healthcare system. In: Analytics, operations, and strategic decision making in the public sector. IGI Global, 2019, 166–186.

[7]   Langfelder P, Horvath S. WGCNA: An R package for weighted correlation network analysis. BMC Bioinform, 2008, 9(1), 559.

[8]   Jones PJ, Mair P, McNally RJ. Visualizing psychological networks: A tutorial in R. Front Psychol, 2018, 9, 1742.

[9]   Dima AL. Scale validation in applied health research: Tutorial for a 6-step R-based psychometrics protocol. Health Psychol Behav Med, 2018, 6(1), 136–161.

[10] Rietveld T, Van Hout R. Statistical techniques for the study of language behaviour. Berlin, Mouton de Gruyter, 1993.

[11] Matsunaga M. How to factor-analyze your data right: Do's, don'ts, and how-to's. Int J Psychol Stud, 2010, 3(1), 97–110.

[12] Brown TA. Confirmatory factor analysis for applied research. 2nd ed. New York, The Guildford Press, 2015.

[13] Child D. The essentials of factor analysis. 2nd ed. London, Cassel Educational Limited, 1990.

[14] Suhr DD Exploratory or confirmatory factor analysis? Proceedings of the 31st Annual SAS? Users Group International Conference. Cary, NC, SAS Institute. 2006.

[15] DeCoster J. Overview of factor analysis, 1998. (Accessed August 10, 2021, at: http://www.stat-help.com/notes.html ().

[16] Snowden A, Stenhouse R, Young J, Carver H, Carver F, Brown N. The relationship between emotional intelligence, previous caring experience and mindfulness in student nurses and midwives: A cross sectional analysis. Nurse Educ Today, 2015, 35(1), 152–158.

[17] Petrides KV. Psychometric properties of the Trait Emotional Intelligence Questionnaire. In: Stough C, Saklofske DH, Parker JD, eds. Advances in the assessment of emotional intelligence. New York, Springer, 2009.
[18] Freudenthaler HH, Neubauer AC, Gabler P, Scherl WG. Testing the Trait Emotional Intelligence Questionnaire (TEIQue) in a German-speaking sample. Pers Individ Differ, 2008, 45, 673–678.
[19] Petrides KV, Furnham A. The role of trait emotional intelligence in a gender-specific model of organizational variables. J Appl Soc Psychol, 2006, 36, 552–569.
[20] Zampetakis LA. Chapter 11: The measurement of trait emotional intelligence with TEIQue-SF: An analysis based on unfolding item response theory models'. In: Härtel CEJ, Ashkanasy NM, Zerbe WJ, eds. Research on emotion in organizations. 2011, vol. 7, 289–315.
[21] Stiglic G, Cilar Budler L, Watson R. Data for: Running a Confirmatory Factor Analysis in R: a step-by-step tutorial, Mendeley Data, V1, 2022; doi: 10.17632/bkh8wtgmkg.1.
[22] Albright JJ. Confirmatory factor analysis using AMOS, LISREL, and MPLUS. The Trustees of Indiana University, 2006.
[23] Salkind NJ. Encyclopedia of research design. vol. 1, Sage, 2010.
[24] Kyriazos TA. Applied psychometrics: Sample size and sample power considerations in factor analysis (EFA, CFA) and SEM in general. Psychology, 2018, 9(08), 2207.
[25] Kaiser HF. A second generation little jiffy. Psychometrika, 1970, 35(4), 401–415.
[26] Brown TA, Moore MT. Confirmatory factor analysis. Handb Struct Equation Model, 2012, 361–379.
[27] Korkmaz S, Goksuluk D, Zararsiz G, An MVN. R package for assessing multivariate normality. R J, 2014, 6(2), 151–162.
[28] Finney SJ, DiStefano C. Non-normal and categorical data in structural equation modeling. In: Hancock GR, Mueller RO, eds. Structural equation modeling: A second course. 2nd ed. Charlotte, NC, Information Age Publishing, 2013, 439–492.
[29] Epskamp S, Cramer AO, Waldorp LJ, Schmittmann VD, Borsboom D. qgraph: Network visualizations of relationships in psychometric data. J Stat Softw, 2012, 48(4), 1–18.
[30] JFJr H, Black WC, Babin BJ, Anderson RE, Tatham RL. Multivariate data analysis. 7th ed. Prentice-Hall, Upper Saddle River, 2010.
[31] Jackson DL, Gillaspy Jr JA, Purc-Stephenson R. Reporting practices in confirmatory factor analysis: An overview and some recommendations. Psychol Methods, 2009, 14(1), 6.
[32] Tabachnick BG, Fidell LS. Using multivariate statistics. 5th ed. Boston, Allyn and Bacon, 2007.
[33] Hu L, Bentler PM. Cutoff criteria for fit indexes in covariance structure analysis: Conventional criteria versus new alternatives. Struct Equation Model, 1999, 6, 1–55.
[34] Tucker LR, Lewis C. A reliability coefficient for maximum likelihood factor analysis. Psychometrika, 1973, 38, 1–10.
[35] Chavez A, Koutentakis D, Liang Y, Tripathy S, Yun J. Identify Statistical Similarities and Differences Between the Deadliest Cancer Types Through Gene Expression. 2019.
[36] Shi D, Maydeu-Olivares A, Rosseel Y. Assessing fit in ordinal factor analysis models: SRMR vs. RMSEA. Struct Equ Model, 2020, 27(1), 1–15.
[37] Grove SK, Gray JR. Understanding nursing research E-book: Building an evidence-based practice. Elsevier Health Sci, 2018.
[38] Narayanan A. A review of eight software packages for structural equation modeling. Am Stat, 2012, 66(2), 129–138.
[39] R Core Team. A Language and Environment for Statistical Computing, 2013. (Accessed August 10, 2021), at: http://www.R-project.org.

[40] Hagen B, Awasoga O, Kellett P, Die O. Evaluation of undergraduate nursing students' attitudes towards statistics courses, before and after a course in applied statistics. Nurse Educ Today, 2013, 33, 949–955.
[41] Ritz C, Streibig JC. Bioassay analysis using R. J Stat Softw, 2005, 125.
[42] Arbuckle JL. IBM SPSS AMOS 20 user's guide. Armonk, IBM Corporation, 2011.
[43] Oberski D. lavaan. survey: An R package for complex survey analysis of structural equation models. J Stat Softw, 2014, 57(1), 1–27.

Index